PMT
The Unrecognised Illness

Judy Lever with
Dr M. Brush and Brian Haynes

NEW ENGLISH LIBRARY/TIMES MIRROR

First published in Great Britain in 1979 by Melbourne House
© 1979 by Judy Lever and Brian Haynes

First NEL Paperback Edition September 1980

NEL Books are published by
New English Library Limited from
Barnard's Inn, Holborn,
London EC1N 2JR.
Made and printed in Great Britain by
Hunt Barnard Printing Ltd.,
Aylesbury, Bucks.

0 450 04766 0

CONTENTS

Acknowledgements

My thanks are due to many people. To David Elstein who, as producer of the 'This Week' programme at Thames Television continually encouraged and supported my interest in PMT; to the team at Thames Television who helped in the making of a 'This Week' programme about PMT; to Dr Katherina Dalton who has always generously given me the benefit of her knowledge; to Charles Vetter who generously gave me the benefit of his experience and who made useful comments on the manuscript; to Professor Ronald Taylor for allowing me access to the extensive research he and his department have undertaken; to Lindsay Harvey who generously allowed me to read her thesis on PMT.

A special thank you must go to the people who worked with me on the book. To the thousands of women who spoke or wrote so frankly about their experience of PMT; to Dr Michael Brush for his patient explanations and careful reading and correction of each draft of the manuscript; to Brian Haynes for his enthusiastic help with the research; to Ian Kestle for adding his touch; to Naomi for her energetic and sympathetic support throughout the preparation and editing of the book and to Roger who subjected my arguments to much helpful debate, corrected my grammar and spelling, kept me at it and would like to think he wrote the best bits.

Judy Lever
1979

Foreword

There is little doubt that for many healthy women at the most active and demanding period of their lives, the physical and emotional changes which occur in the week or so before menstruation constitute a great burden and sometimes a hazard to their personal relationships. For many who suffer from such pre menstrual distress the greatest problem is a lack of understanding of the physical processes which cause the mental changes. There is often a deep fear that there is a true and severe psychiatric abnormality.

It has been our experience that explanation of the pre menstrual syndrome goes a long way to reassuring sufferers, while the further knowledge that help is available is an equal comfort. This book is one of the most helpful I have read from the point of view of explaining things to sufferers – among whom it must be mentioned are many husbands and families of the women concerned. I think that in itself it will have a real therapeutic value.

R. W. Taylor
Professor of Gynaecology
St Thomas's Hospital Medical School
London

Introduction

Millions of women suffer from it. It is painful, depressing, frightening, sometimes devastating. It affects women all over the world, in primitive as well as civilised societies, women who are placid or highly strung, the rich and the poor. It has been called the world's commonest illness. Yet, until very recently, it was scarcely recognised as a genuine illness.

It is pre menstrual tension – PMT for short. Estimates vary, but it is believed that more than three quarters of all women suffer some of the symptoms of PMT. For some, the symptoms are only a nuisance, causing two or three days of mild discomfort. But for over a third of women the symptoms are severe and can last from a few days to two weeks before each period. These are distressing and disruptive enough to need treatment.

The consequences of PMT are staggering. Surveys have shown that half of all accidents occurring to women at home, at work, or on the road, occur during the pre menstrual week. PMT lies behind female hospital admissions, female criminal offences and over half of all suicide attempts by women. Sportswomen dread important events falling during their pre menstrual week. Women are more likely to batter their babies or physically attack their husbands. Women with drinking problems drink more heavily or relapse more readily. PMT can destroy a woman's personal life and hamper her career.

Yet for years PMT has been misunderstood. Doctors were baffled by it, particularly by the variety of symptoms. They believed that it was 'all in the mind' or they put it down as an inevitable part of the menstrual cycle. Women complaining of the most common symptoms – headaches, swelling, aches and pains, tension, lethargy, irritability, depression – often found their visits to the doctor a frustrating and humiliating experience.

They were told: 'Pull yourself together' or 'It is all part of being a woman'. Or they were given useless remedies which attempted to treat the symptoms without touching the cause.

Scientific evidence has now firmly established that PMT has a physical cause. In those women who suffer from it there is a malfunction in the production of hormones during the menstrual cycle, in particular the female hormone, progesterone. This upsets the normal working of the menstrual cycle and produces the unpleasant symptoms of PMT.

As a result of this discovery, treatments have been devised which are simple, safe and remarkably successful. More than three-quarters of women who have been treated appear to be completely cured or helped to the point where their symptoms are easily bearable.

This book gives you the facts about PMT. We explain the causes and the symptoms and we bring you up to date on the cure. We tell you what the doctor can do for you and suggest ways you can help yourself. And we draw on the experiences of the thousands of women who have written to us, called us or spoken to us to try to explain what it is like to suffer from PMT and how much better life can be after treatment.

Answering your Questions

Ever since I started to write this book, I have been bombarded with questions about PMT. Friends, acquaintances, colleagues, people I bump into have all wanted to clear up points that bothered them. You may be the same. So here, for quick reference, are the questions that came up most often, with the answers I gave to them. You will find that most of the questions are answered in more detail in the book.

Q How can I tell if I am suffering from PMT? What are the symptoms?

A There are a wide variety of symptoms. The most common are headaches, painful breasts, weight gain due to water retention, mood swings, irritability, lethargy and depression. There is a full check-list of symptoms on Page 110. But the key to whether or not you are suffering from PMT is not so much the symptoms you get as **when** you get them. If your symptoms occur every month, or almost every month, in the days before your period, and stop as soon as your period starts, or shortly after, then you are probably suffering from PMT. The best way to find out is to keep a menstrual chart for at least two months, so that you can see if there is a definite pattern to your symptoms. You will find a menstrual chart and instructions on how to fill it in, on Page 107.

Q Why do I get PMT?

A Scientific evidence so far indicates that you get PMT when the hormones controlling your menstrual cycle are out of balance. This can happen for a variety of reasons, which we look at in Chapter Three.

Q Will my symptoms be the same every month?

A You will probably find that your symptoms are more or less the same every month, and that you suffer from several at the same time. But sometimes one symptom may not occur at all, or a symptom – like headaches for instance – may be more severe in some months than in others.

Q If I get symptoms some months but not others, can I really have PMT?

A PMT is notable for the way in which the symptoms recur every, or nearly every month. If you go for several months without symptoms the chances are that you are not suffering from PMT. Keep a menstrual chart (see Page 107). This will show you the pattern and regularity of your symptoms.

Q I get some of the symptoms of PMT at any time of the month, not just before my periods. Why?

A Because you are not suffering from PMT! As you will realise, none of the symptoms of PMT are specific to PMT. They can be unrelated to your period, and of course men can suffer from most of them too. You are only suffering from PMT if your symptoms occur regularly in the days before your period.

Q I have been told that PMT is 'all in the mind'. Is that true?

A No, it is not. Studies have largely disproved the idea that only neurotic or highly strung women suffer from PMT. PMT is basically a physical problem. But women who have psychological difficulties may have an increased chance of suffering from the psychological symptoms of PMT.

Q Will treatment really help?

A Yes! Over three-quarters of all the women who have received one of the treatments in this book appear to have been completely cured or have gained considerable relief from their symptoms. It is a question of finding the treatment that suits you best. Once you do, there is every chance that you will find relief from PMT.

Q How long does treatment take to work?

A Some women get almost immediate relief from their symptoms. Others take a little time to react, or find that some of their symptoms persist after others have disappeared. It may take time to establish the treatment that works best for you, or to get the dosage exactly right.

14

Q How long do I have to continue treatment?

A Usually treatment lasts for between six to nine months. But some women find that their symptoms recur once they stop treatment. If that happens to you, you may need to continue treatment for longer, perhaps reducing your dosage gradually over the months. Your doctor should know what is likely to bring you the greatest relief. I know one woman who has been taking natural progesterone each month before her symptoms are due for nearly 15 years, with apparently no ill effects.

Q Can I lead an ordinary life during treatment?

A Yes. None of the main treatments in this book need affect your life in any way except, I hope, to relieve you of PMT.

Q I have been prescribed tranquillisers. Do they do any good?

A Tranquillisers are **not** a treatment for PMT, and in some cases actually make some of the symptoms worse. See Chapter Eleven for details.

Q Are there any harmful side effects of treatment?

A The vitamin and hormone treatments that we mention do not appear, in all the research that has been done on them to date, to have any harmful side effects. Some women occasionally suffer minor menstrual changes on the hormone treatment. Another treatment, the powerful drug bromocryptine, has more unpleasant side effects, though they have not been shown to be dangerous, and this is really a 'last resort' treatment if all else fails. We look at treatments and their side effects in detail in Chapter Eleven.

Q Can I help myself without a doctor?

A It all depends on the severity of your symptoms. If they are relatively mild, you may be able to manage them yourself. And if you do not want to go to a doctor, or do not want hormone tablets, you can follow the advice in Chapter Ten, or try the vitamin treatment in Chapter Eleven for yourself. But if your symptoms are very severe, you probably need your doctor's help.

Q My symptoms are uncomfortable but I couldn't call them severe. Is it worth getting treatment?

A You are the best judge of that. If your symptoms bother you, then you probably want to do something about them. The advice in Chapter Ten may be enough to help you but, if not, there is no reason why you should not go to see your doctor.

O I do not have PMT yet. Am I likely to get it?

A I hope not! Often PMT begins at puberty or soon after, though it may get worse as you get older. But some women find that they only start to suffer from PMT after the birth of their first baby. If you have already had children and do not suffer from PMT, the chances are very good indeed that you never will.

Q Can I outgrow PMT?

A PMT tends to get worse, rather than better, with age, so I doubt that you will outgrow it. But I hope that, after reading this book, you will find ways to make it much better, or to get rid of it completely.

Q Can I suffer from PMT if I have had a hysterectomy?

A Yes. A hysterectomy removes either the womb alone or the womb and ovaries. If you still have one or both of your ovaries, the cyclical hormone changes can still continue, even though there is now no response from the womb. If you suffered from PMT before the operation, it is quite likely that your symptoms will recur after the operation, although you may get a few good months before they do. And there is also some evidence that women are more likely to suffer from depression after a hysterectomy, or that their PMT symptoms can be more severe. Occasionally doctors suggest a hysterectomy as treatment for PMT. This is ridiculous. If that is the only reason for having a hysterectomy, you have every right to refuse the operation, and you would be far better off trying one of the treatments in this book.

Q I have passed the menopause but I still get some of the symptoms of PMT. Could PMT treatments help?

A No. The menopause is a gradual process in which the production of the hormones associated with menstruation diminishes and the ovaries and womb shrink. At the point when your periods stop completely, even if some of your symptoms seem like those of PMT, they are no longer directly connected with your period, their cause is different and so they need different treatment. However, if you are going through the transition to the menopause, Vitamin B6 may help you. (See page 131 for details).

Q I have been to my doctor many times and he does not seem willing or able to help. What can I do?

A Times are gradually changing, but some doctors are still very unsympathetic to women with PMT. If your doctor's treatment has not helped you, there are a number of things you can do. You could change doctors. Or you could ask, as you have a right to do, to be referred for the opinion of an endocrinologist, who will be attached to a hospital. Or you could seek out a specialist PMT clinic. More are opening up all the time, either independently or attached to hospitals, so there is a chance you may find one near you. And, of course, there are a variety of ways you can help yourself until you find a suitable doctor. (See Chapter Ten and Appendix).

Chapter One

The Physical Symptoms

You wake up one morning and it is as if the sun has gone in suddenly. You know, even before it has started, that today is going to be a bad day. You feel heavy and bloated and your head aches.

As the day wears on, your headache gets worse and you feel increasingly miserable. The next three days are hell. You get that can't-be-bothered-to-do-anything feeling. You are irritable and depressed by turns. Next day, your period starts and it is as if the clouds have lifted. You are your usual self again.

If that sounds like you, then you may well be suffering from pre menstrual tension. The first thing you should know about PMT is that it can affect you in a great many ways. There are a wide variety of symptoms, some physical, some psychological, some more common than others. You may suffer several, or you may only have one or two, some may be relatively mild, others may be quite severe.

Exactly how PMT affects **you** depends on your particular physical make-up, personality and circumstances. You may, for example, come from a family with a history of head-aches, so headaches may be one of your worst symptoms. Or you may work at a job that puts particular strain on your back muscles, so back ache may be your worst symptom. You will notice as you read on that none of the symptoms I mention are specific to PMT. Some women suffer from them but do not have PMT. And, of course, many men can have them too. **So it is not what symptoms you have which gives you the clue to whether you have PMT. It is when you get them.**

Do the symptoms recur with miserable regularity every, or nearly every month?

Do you usually get several symptoms at the same time?

Do you find that things you may suffer at any time, like headaches or lack of energy, are much worse in the week or so before your periods?

Do you suddenly feel better as soon as your period starts?

Do you have at least one good week each month when you cannot understand how you could have felt so down in the bad days?

If you answered a silent 'yes' to most of these questions, you are very probably suffering from PMT. But it is quite likely you answered 'I don't know' because you have never really stopped to think whether or not your symptoms occur just before your period is due. You have probably never even thought of your headaches or depression as 'symptoms' anyway. Many women do not realise that there is a more or less regular **pattern** to their symptoms, that they occur at the same time each month. Many doctors, too, miss the pattern because they look just at the symptoms and not at their timing.

Carol, a 30 year old secretary, went to her doctor time and again complaining of headaches and depression. He gave her tranquillisers which made her feel 'dopey' but did nothing to take away the pain and misery. One day, suspecting PMT, he suggested to Carol that she keep a check on when her symptoms occurred. In fact, Carol had been keeping a diary for years, in which she recorded rows with boyfriends, days she felt particularly depressed, days when she felt really good . . . and the day her period started. She looked back through the diary and found, to her amazement, that her symptoms always occurred just before her period was due.

If you are not sure when your symptoms occur, it is a

good idea to keep a menstrual chart for two or three months to find out. We show you how in Chapter Nine.

* * *

Once, most doctors believed that the **whole** problem was psychological, that it was 'all in the mind'. You were 'neurotic' and that was why you had these headaches. You were 'highly strung' and so complained over trivial ailments that other people weathered without a murmur.

But things are changing now. Dr Anthony Clare, a British psychiatrist, has shown in studies conducted over the last three years that a large proportion of women suffering PMT do not respond in the way one would expect them to if the cause was only psychological. **Research in Britain, Europe and the United States has shown that PMT has a very definite cause,** with clear physical as well as psychological symptoms.

I should say at this stage that there is no easy dividing line between the physical and psychological symptoms and they are often intertwined. For instance, your body tissues may retain extra water before your period, so that you put on weight and feel bloated. This can make you feel depressed or lethargic – the physical leading to the psychological. On the other hand, feelings of stress can lead to headaches or migraine – the psychological leading to the physical. Not surprisingly, with PMT most sufferers experience several of the symptoms together. Nevertheless, in the rest of this chapter I shall deal only with the physical symptoms of PMT.

If none of these apply to you, you can skip these symptoms and go on to Chapter Two.

* * *

Water retention (Oedema)

You may find that you put on anything from four to seven pounds in weight just before your period. Some women go up as much as fourteen pounds. This is not a coincidence or caused simply because you have been eating or drinking too much. What is happening is that your tissues and cells retain more water than usual under the influence of complicated hormonal changes taking place in your body at this time of the month (more about those in Chapter Three).

Normally this water is lost naturally through sweating or urination but, just before your period, it can collect and stay in your body instead of passing to your kidneys for excretion. The water often collects in particular parts of the body, exactly where depending on your individual make-up. Favourite places are ankles, legs, fingers, abdomen and breasts.

Many women find that their rings do not fit or their shoes become tight and uncomfortable. Others notice that their stomachs stick out embarrassingly and their clothes do not fit properly any more. One woman described herself as 'blowing up like a balloon'. Like lots of other women, she kept special 'fat' clothes and a larger size bra for this time of the month.

If the water collects in your ankles and feet, you may find it hard to stand still for any length of time. You may also feel faint, and desperately try to find something to lean against to stop you falling over.

Sometimes the walls of your intestine store water at this time and become 'water logged'. Some of this water may be drawn from the bowel passageway and this can make you constipated, increasing the heavy, bloated feeling.

The effects of water retention are probably worst of all when the water collects in parts of your body where there

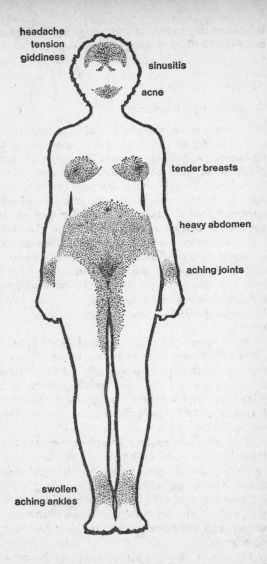

How the physical symptoms can affect you

is little room for the tissues to stretch. If water collects in the eyeball, for instance, the increased pressure on the eye can be very painful. If it collects in the bony skull, it may help to cause, or increase, a headache or migraine. Annoyingly, too, cells that have recently been injured are also more likely to become waterlogged, so that if you recently broke your ankle it is likely that this will 'play up' for a few months afterwards.

It is not surprising that water retention can be very depressing, because it makes you feel heavy, bloated and uncomfortable. The effect is more devastating if you are on a diet. Suddenly all your hard work and self sacrifice seem useless. Many women feel 'Oh to hell with it, since I'm so fat today anyway I might as well eat' and tuck into all the forbidden foods that they had denied themselves until then.

The fact to remember is that, as soon as your period starts, your tissues will release the excess fluid and the water weight will begin to melt away. You may notice that you sweat more, or find yourself passing water more frequently around this time of the month as your body returns to its usual size again.

Tender Breasts

Painful, swollen breasts are one of the most common symptoms of PMT. Women who only suffer mild PMT often find that this is the worst, and occasionally their only symptom.

A friend of mine is a good example of that. She had never thought about PMT, but one day she confided in me that she was very worried about her breasts.

'I don't know what's wrong with them but sometimes, for no reason that I can see, they become much larger and very painful. Even an affectionate hug from my husband is agony. Just as I start to think I will go to the doctor this time, they get better and I feel as if I'm making a fuss over nothing.'

I mentioned PMT and suggested that she keep a record of the days when her breasts were swollen and the day her

23

period started. Sure enough, her breasts swelled regularly just before her period. She had never noticed the connection. She went to her doctor, who was sympathetic, and gave her appropriate treatment which made all the difference.

Excess water in the breast tissues is partly to blame for the pain and swelling, but it is not the whole story. The hormonal changes that take place at this time can have an effect on the amount of blood flowing through the skin and underlying tissues of the breast. Some women are more sensitive to this than others.

Food cravings

It is well known that many women get unusual and sudden food cravings when they are pregnant. In much the same way, you may get cravings for certain foods in the week or so before your period. You will probably find that you want sweet or high carbohydrate things like cakes, chocolate, ice cream or fizzy drinks.

Jane, a 35 year old hairdresser, admits that she raids the kitchen and eats a whole loaf of bread in one day, instead of her usual careful two slices. Sarah, a 19 year old typist, who is normally very figure conscious, can get through two bars of chocolate in one afternoon just before her period.

There may be a simple psychological reason why you want to eat something you are fond of. If you are feeling miserable, food can be a great comforter. You think: 'I feel so depressed I might as well cheer myself up with something I like – at least it will take my mind off everything else for a while.'

But another reason for these cravings can be a drop in the amount of sugar in your blood. Normally, it stays between 70 to 105 milligrams per 100 millilitres of blood, though it may go up to as much as 170 milligrams after you have eaten a meal with something sweet in it. If the level drops below 70 milligrams, the nerve cells in your body are starved of vital nourishment and this can produce a variety of unpleasant symptoms. Recent research has shown that the hormone changes that take place before your period can lower the amount of sugar in your blood with the result that you need to top it up, or it may increase the amount of sugar you need. Your body signals this and you respond by desiring sweet things that would act quickly to raise your blood sugar level.

Knowing the reason for your cravings does not necessarily make them easier to bear, particularly if you are on a diet. You may find that all your will power suddenly deserts you at this time of the month and, as you fill up on all the fattening forbidden foods, you put on weight. And, unlike the water weight, this weight will not melt away as your period arrives. It will turn into fat and stay with you – at least until, feeling stronger again, you start dieting and the pattern is repeated the following month.

Treating your PMT will help. And there are also ways you can help yourself. In Chapter Ten we look at the whole question of diet: what to do in the bad times, and how to stick to a diet all the time.

Headaches

Headaches come in a variety of types, and pre menstrual headaches are no exception. Sometimes they start suddenly, and are immediately very painful. At other times they build up gradually, creeping upon you over the course of a day or more. Some headaches have obvious causes, others are a mystery.

One reason for headaches, at any time, not just before your period, is spasm of the blood vessels in your head, which expand and contract in reaction to an upset in your nervous system. It may be upset for all sorts of reasons and one of these is the hormonal changes of PMT.

Stress can be another 'trigger' which sets off a headache. You may be very anxious about something, or very excited, and this can set off the chain reaction to a headache. As you will know if you suffer, PMT can be enough on its own to have this effect. But if it is coupled with extra stresses, the

25

chances of a bad headache, or tension headache as it is known, are obviously much increased.

If you get this sort of headache, you will probably feel a throbbing pain and a tightness in your forehead. Several women describe it as a 'steel band tightening round my head'.

However, you might find that you get a tremendous pain above your eyes and in your cheeks, when it hurts if you turn your head suddenly, or bend over. In this case, you are probably suffering from a headache caused by water retention, when the cells in the entrance to your sinus swell and block the nasal passage. This can cause pressure to build up, and make it hard to breathe.

Jo, a 34 year old advertising copywriter, gets two types of headaches.

'The first type of headache attacks the right side of my head right down my face and lasts three days. In these days I don't eat at all. I lie down but cannot sleep. The pain is just indescribable. The second type attacks my left side – I feel the nerve inside my mouth being pulled. That sort lasts for a week, and tablets don't seem to help.'

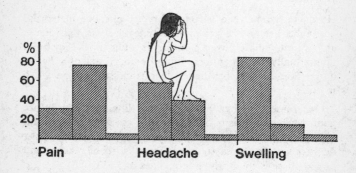

Timing of physical symptoms, before, during and after period.
(Percentage indicates the percentage of women who suffer moderate or severe symptoms.)

26

Headaches are unpredictable. Sometimes they respond to tablets, at least to start with, sometimes they do not. Some headaches last a day, some take as long as a week to go away. Pre menstrual headaches are often more persistent and more painful than occasional headaches you may get at other times of the month. In fact, this is something you will probably notice with PMT. Problems which may be mild at other times of the month are worse in the week before your period.

Migraine

Pre menstrual tension sometimes leads to migraine. It often develops out of an 'ordinary' pre menstrual headache. It starts by attacking one side of your head, with a constant, violent throbbing pain, when your head feels as if it is going to burst. As the migraine develops, it becomes more diffuse and spreads right through your skull, while the throbbing gives way to a persistent ache.

Migraines often last longer than ordinary headaches – anything from a few hours to several days. Sufferers may see bright or flashing lights just before an attack, or feel dizzy and sick, or complain of numbness and pins and needles down one side. You may even actually vomit.

Brenda, a shop assistant, gets bad migraine nearly every month, a few days before her period.

'I suffer terrible migraine, with loss of vision, flashing lights and dizziness. If I go to a crowded store my head starts to spin, my knees and hands shake. I know people are staring at me and I feel so ashamed.'

As with ordinary pre menstrual headaches, painkillers can perhaps help for a while, but sometimes they leave the pain untouched. Some women go to extraordinary lengths to try to rid themselves of the persistent, nagging pain. Ursula, an executive in a consumer organisation, admits that she has banged her head against a brick wall in desperation. Maureen, a student nurse, says: 'I have dug my fingernails into my face and put a hot water bottle on my face, all to counteract the pain of migraine and neuralgia.'

27

One reason for this, as with ordinary headaches, is changes in the flow of blood through the blood vessels in the brain, due to hormonal change. Other reasons are less clear. Water retention for example may play a small part if water collects in your skull.

Lowered blood sugar level is another suspect. As we saw earlier, lowered blood sugar level can be a problem for PMT sufferers. If you feel sick and distraught because of PMT you may skip a meal because you just do not feel like eating. This may well make matters worse.

It might be that your family has a history of migraine attacks. In the normal course of events that does not mean that you will automatically suffer too. What it does mean is that, if you suffer from PMT, then one of your symptoms may well be migraine.

Aches and Pains

Aches and pains are one of the most common nuisances of PMT. You wake up one morning, a few days before your period, and feel stiff. Then a dull ache begins in your back or your knees or ankles which continues to annoy you for the next few days until, miraculously it seems, it disappears as soon as your period starts.

Sometimes the aches are in your shoulders, or hands, feet or hips. They are usually not very painful, but they are a nagging irritant you can well do without. The reason for them may be water gathering in those places, or it may simply be that your muscles are stiff and unrelaxed because you are feeling tense generally.

If these pains do not go away once your period starts, you may well have a more serious condition that needs checking. As with all symptoms, it is tempting to blame PMT for everything. You should always check that they really do occur only before your period, regularly each or nearly every month, and that you have at least one week when you do not get any aches or pains at all.

Clumsiness and lack of co-ordination

One of my biggest surprises when I first started to find out about PMT was that clumsiness is one of the symptoms. It sounds so odd. But once I started talking to women about it, it was clear that they really do become clumsier and more unco-ordinated at the pre menstrual time.

Like them, you may find you suddenly seem to drop things more often or bump into furniture around the house. Sonia, a housewife, reckons that 'we scarcely have a cup left with a handle on any more, thanks to me. Now my husband does the washing up for the days before my period!' Many women find they tend to burn themselves while cooking or cut themselves more frequently.

It is tempting to think that these women are just naturally clumsy anyway, but studies to test women for co-ordination at general tasks and in sport, for example, show that there definitely is a difference for some women in the pre menstrual days. But nobody is sure exactly why this is. Many doctors think it is caused by lack of concentration, bred of tension. When you are feeling edgy and tense, 'at odds with yourself', you may find it harder to concentrate and your mind will keep drifting off on to other things.

Tension can also make your muscles stiff and unsupple, so that your grip is not as firm as usual and you do not move freely and easily. Women who play a lot of sport and who also suffer from PMT, sometimes notice that they do not give their best performances and make annoying, unforced errors. We look at lack of co-ordination and accident proneness in detail in Chapter Seven.

* * *

We have looked at the ways PMT is most likely to affect you. But besides these more common physical symptoms, there are a number of others which are less usual but do strike some women before their periods.

One of these is **asthma.** Pre menstrual asthma often begins acutely in the middle of the night, continues for hours or days and then suddenly stops when menstruation starts. An asthma allergy clinic in Britain found that about one third of all the women of child-bearing age had a tendency to pre menstrual asthma attacks, especially around puberty and when reaching the menopause.

Although asthma is often an allergic reaction, pre menstrual asthma seems to be caused by water retention in the cells and tissues in the smaller tubes of the lung. They become swollen and so restrict the flow of air into the air sacs.

Another serious physical illness that can sometimes be related to PMT is **epilepsy**. Doctors have found a certain number of women who suffer epileptic attacks only in their pre menstrual week. Often these attacks follow increasingly severe headaches and a build up of tension. If you suffer like this only before your period, you should find that treating your PMT can completely eliminate the attacks and you will not need to take anti-convulsant drugs any more.

Some women suffer eye infections like **conjunctivitis** or **glaucoma**, a disease of the eye characterised by raised pressure in the eyeball. The Institute of Opthalmology in London found that 89% of women suffering from closed angle glaucoma also suffered from PMT, and 60% of the women experienced glaucoma in the days prior to their periods. It is possible, though by no means certain, that water retention is at least partly to blame for the fact that these two problems, epilepsy and glaucoma, occur pre menstrually, when swollen tissues and cells increase the pressure in the head or eyes and trigger an attack.

Acne and **cold sores** can all be symptoms of pre menstrual tension. You may notice that you get spotty before your period or your skin becomes pink and blotchy, but this fades once your period starts.

Oddly, perhaps, **spontaneous bruising**, when bruises appear on your body although you have not suffered a blow, has also been associated with PMT, though it is not very common. On page 110 we give a check-list of most of the symptoms that may be related to PMT.

Finally, a note of caution. You may have already decided

that you are definitely suffering from PMT because you have suffered from some of the symptoms described in this chapter. Good! That means that you are aware that PMT exists. But the wide variety of symptoms, and the fact that they are not specific to PMT, can be misleading. There is one easy way to find out if you really are suffering from PMT: keep a menstrual chart for three months to see when your symptoms occur. That is the true indicator of PMT. We show you how in Chapter Nine.

Dr Dalton, who has studied PMT for over 30 years, tells the story of a girl who had been sent to her because the girl's doctor suspected that her regular migraine attacks were caused by PMT. Dr Dalton found that the girl's attacks came at **fortnightly** intervals, originally on Tuesdays but later on Thursdays. On checking the girl's menstrual chart it was clear that the attacks were not connected with her period at all. In fact, it turned out that she used to go direct to her hairdresser after work on Tuesdays, after only a snack lunch, and then on Thursdays when her favourite hairdresser changed her night. The girl's migraine attacks were triggered by not eating, and had absolutely no connection with her periods.

Chapter Two

The Psychological Symptoms

'I feel it is not me that is in possession of my body. I change personality, which is very difficult for the people I live and work with. I've tried, every month I try. I say "this month it's going to be different, I'm not going to let it get hold of me". But when it actually comes to it something chemical happens to me. I can't control it, it just happens.'

If your ankles swell, your breasts are sore and you have a blinding headache, people will probably be sympathetic. After all, there is obviously something wrong with you. But if you are snappy and short tempered, or keep bursting into tears for no apparent reason, they will probably give you short shrift.

You may yourself be bewildered by your behaviour. Perhaps the last thing you would think of is that it can have anything to do with your periods. Yet psychological symptoms like these are very common, and are often the worst aspect of PMT.

As we mentioned in Chapter One, **it is very likely that you will get both psychological and physical symptoms**, which intertwine. But some women only have psychological symptoms, and this may make the connection with your period even harder to detect.

Tension

The word 'tension' was used to describe the whole illness in

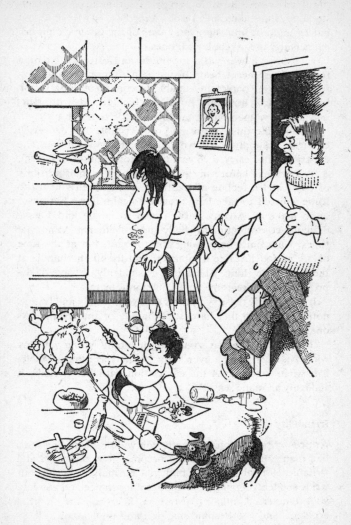

the days before the wide variety of symptoms was understood, and the name has stuck. As it happens tension does indeed underlie and aggravate many of the other symptoms, particularly the psychological ones.

Tension is a worrying, miserable and often frightening feeling. Your heart beats faster, you cannot breathe, you feel a surge of panic, and unable to cope. You long to ask for help but do not know how. You feel 'at odds with yourself' as one woman put it, unable to settle to anything.

Feeling like this, you often grow irritable and depressed by turns, or simply flop down and give up on everything. The experience of Lesley, a 26 year old factory worker, is typical:

'A few days before my period I get an increasing sense of panic and a feeling of tightness inside, when you try to force yourself to take long breaths to calm down but never quite make it. All my nerves seem to jangle and I have difficulty co-ordinating my body and movements. At normal times, I am quite easy going and tolerant, but at the time of my period I'm like a monster, and fly off the handle at the least little thing. Then, just as suddenly, a wave of depression sweeps over me, and I burst into tears.'

It is probably these symptoms that your family and friends notice most and find hardest to handle or understand. As one man told me:

'I thought there was something mentally wrong with my wife. And I think she even thought she was a bit unstable. But when we realised the connection with her periods, it suddenly all made sense!'

Irritability

As pre-period tension builds up, you will probably find that, like many PMT sufferers, you become short tempered and irritable. Trivial incidents that you normally take in your stride suddenly assume tremendous importance and you lose your temper. A minor frustration, a cross word, a little accident, and you become snappish and unpleasant.

It is hardly surprising really. If you are feeling tense and your head aches, it is much harder to cope with run-of-the-mill worries that crop up. Frustration at feeling so helpless can easily lead to temper. The temptation is to lash out and blame it all on something or someone else.

Jane, a journalist, found this problem:

'Something seems to snap in my head. I go from a normal state of mind to anger, when I'm really nasty. Usually I'm very even tempered but in these times it is as if someone else, not me, is doing all this and it is very frightening.'

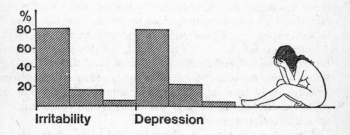

Timing of psychological symptoms, before, during and after period.
(Percentage indicates percentage of women who suffer moderate or severe symptoms.)

Sometimes irritability can grow to become fierce temper. Sharon frightens herself by the violence of her feelings:

'When my black moods descend, I have to struggle to continue to be polite at work and when I get home I let go. I get fits of uncontrollable temper when I throw myself on the floor and tear out my hair.'

Some women turn this aggression outwards, and lash out, usually at those closest to them. Sheila, a 40 year old housewife with two children puts it like this:

'There is such a thin line between screaming vile abuse and doing actual bodily harm sometimes. All my adult life I've suffered from PMT, completely unable to control my vile bad temper, screaming and swearing at my husband, hitting and shaking the children. When it is over I'm left with a terrible feeling of guilt until the next time.'

35

Sadly, some women do cross that thin line and lash out viciously, seriously injuring their husbands or children. The problems of women who batter their families and friends are treated in more detail in Chapters Five and Six.

Depression

Feeling weepy and miserable is another very common symptom. 'Suddenly the world looks black' or 'It is as if a cloud has descended' is how many women describe it. You may find that tears are very close to the surface and you suddenly start crying over stupid, trivial little things.

Often, you are not deeply depressed, but you just do not feel your usual cheerful self. You cannot seem to shake off the sense that nothing you do seems right, and problems you would usually take in your stride, assume miserable importance. Barbara, a 26 year old mother of a small son, finds it disconcerting.

'I only have to lose something like the sugar when I'm baking a cake for instance, and that's it – I burst into tears and sob for minutes on end. I know it frightens my son but there is nothing I can do to stop myself.'

Again, it seems that your hormones are responsible. If the delicate balance of hormones in your body is upset, then your emotional balance is upset also. The brain is intimately linked with the hormonal mechanisms which control your menstrual cycle (which we look at in detail in Chapter Three) so it is not surprising that your physical and emotional well-being are so closely interwoven.

If pre menstrual depression coincides with other problems you are facing, like difficulties at work, or trouble with one of your children, or separation from your husband or boyfriend, then the depression can deepen and become unrelenting. Serious depression like this can have a devastating effect on you and everyone around you.

Sally, who has suffered from PMT for ten years, finds that depression is her most disturbing symptom.

'Sometimes the depression is so bad that I want to die. I feel the only solution is to kill myself. I know this sounds silly and melodramatic but when you get to the state I do it seems the only way out.'

Sally is not unusual. Surveys have shown that suicide attempts by women are much more likely in the pre menstrual week. We look at the serious affects of depression in detail in Chapter Eight.

Lethargy

Sometimes it is a real effort even to get out of bed. You may feel that you just 'cannot be bothered' to do the housework, look after the children or get on with your work at the office. One woman admitted that, when she is feeling like this, she gets up to see her husband and children off to work and school and then creeps straight back upstairs to bed again. If you are naturally energetic or tidy, then you may surprise or shock yourself with the sudden change in personality that overtakes you. Joan, a 38 year old mother of three, is like that:

'I'm usually so houseproud, but just before my period I get into a couldn't-care-less mood and become a real – well, there's only one word for it – a slut. I don't do the housework, I don't cook, I just wander round the house moping. Of course, as soon as the mood lifts, I feel so ashamed of myself and rush round the house wondering how I could have been so stupid. But, three weeks later, no matter how hard I try, the same thing happens all over again.'

Wyn, a business woman I know, who is strikingly energetic normally, admits that her work is affected:

'I have to make an extra effort to get through the day. Whenever a problem comes up, I get this terrible temptation to push it aside and go to sleep instead. I have even dozed off on occasion. Inevitably, my colleagues notice. They'll say, "What's got into you? You're usually so energetic but today you're like a sack of potatoes!"'

It is not too clear what causes lethargy, and though I am classing it as a psychological symptom (in common with many doctors who have studied PMT) it can also have a physical basis. It is possible, for example, that the drop in blood sugar level we mentioned earlier may contribute to tiredness. There is also often a slight imbalance of sodium and potassium in the blood of PMT sufferers and this could be a factor too.

But it seems very likely that lethargy is primarily a psychological response to depression and stress. Psychologists often come across people who complain of feeling tired all the time and retreat to bed for long periods during the day. This can be an extreme way in which distressed or disturbed people avoid confronting difficult situations. Sleeping puts off the evil moment when they have to do something about these problems, and tiredness provides the perfect excuse for inaction. What is more, they really feel tired, so they do not realise the complicated tricks their mind and body are playing.

Pre menstrual lethargy seems to be a milder form of the same thing. To be energetic, you need to feel strong, decisive – making decisions, striding out, being positive. If you are feeling headachy and depressed it is easier to retreat to bed or an armchair rather than face problems as they arise and consider what to do next.

It is ironical though, that you may find that just before PMT hits you, you become very energetic and active, cleaning the house, working harder at the office, keen to go out and see friends. Women often notice this burst of energy at mid-cycle. But then, a day or two later, you become listless and lethargic, hardly wanting to move. Your family or friends, not realising the real cause of the lethargy, will tell you that you have 'brought it on yourself' by doing too much during your energetic phase and getting over-tired. In fact, it is much more likely that the feelings I have described above are beginning to take over.

Sudden mood swings

You may already have noticed how the 'mood symptoms we have been describing frequently seem to strike suddenly, unexpectedly. One minute you are laughing, the next you are in tears. Something trivial can instantly send you from cheerful tolerance into a seething fury.

Such sudden swings of mood can be very frightening because they take you, as well as your family and friends, completely by surprise. You feel out of control, as if your body and mind are acting independently and you have no say in what you do. Jane, the journalist I mentioned earlier, finds her sudden changes of mood very hard to live with.

'I seem to spend the six or seven days before my period swinging from depression to anger and back again. I'll suddenly start to cry because my hair looks awful, and then my boyfriend will come in and I'll immediately jump down his throat over nothing at all. Inevitably the row ends with me in tears again. It seems so ridiculous talking about it now, but no matter what I do it goes on happening.'

One consolation is that the symptoms I have been describing only happen once a month. If you can see a pattern in your behaviour it helps you and everyone around you to realise that this is not how you are all the time. You have not suddenly become a depressive, irritable harridan. Complicated physical processes in your body account for the temporary changes in your personality. Many women describe themselves as 'a sort of Jekyll and Hyde', most of the time capable, loving and able to cope and then suddenly quite the reverse.

For centuries many men, including doctors (and too many women) have believed that the psychological symptoms I have described here are characteristic simply of being a woman. They totally failed to distinguish between minor mood variations, which are quite usual and normal, and which affect men, of course, and the severe symptoms that some women get before their periods. Women, so the theory goes, are by nature erratic and unpredictable, liable to sudden changes of mood at any moment.

Such myths die hard. Their presence lingers even in the minds of doctors today, who often still refuse to recognise that they are dealing with uncharacteristic behaviour which betrays an underlying illness, and this accounts for much of the lack of understanding or help women find in the surgery.

CASE HISTORY: STELLA

To see how the common physical and psychological symptoms can affect one person, here in some detail is the story of Stella. She is 37 years old, married with two children aged six and three.

She used to work as a medical secretary but gave up when she first became pregnant. Her pre menstrual problems started after the birth of her first daughter.

'It was about two months after my daughter was born that I first noticed anything wrong. I started to put on weight about ten days before my period was due. It was as if I was being pumped up like a balloon. I could feel my legs, fingers and then my whole body get bigger. At first I don't think I realised that my weight gain was anything to do with my period. It just seemed to come and go so I thought it was my lack of will power.

'I bought one dress to fit me when I was fat. I would not buy any more because it was a sort of punishment to myself. If I had put on weight I would have to suffer, and anyway I would be good and lose weight tomorrow.

'I felt very sick, too, but I would still rush out and buy myself biscuits and bottles of lemonade. I'd eat a whole packet of biscuits at one go sometimes. Of course, that meant that I really did put on weight and I gradually got fatter and fatter. At my worst, I was 198 pounds. I shudder to think of it now.

'I became very withdrawn and did not want to go out of the house and be seen. I just wanted to go away and hide. I think if I could have found a big hole I would have jumped into it. I was actually afraid of bumping into friends in case they laughed at me and when I went to fetch my eldest daughter from school, or if I went out shopping. I'd rush to get it over with as soon as possible. It got so bad that if I even caught sight of myself in a shop window I'd become depressed and start to cry.

'I think the depression was the worst part. I would sit at home some days for hours at a time, crying without knowing why. I didn't feel like doing anything. I wouldn't play with the children, I wouldn't go out with my husband, I wouldn't ask friends round. Actually I'm rather a jolly person and enjoy going out and being sociable. My husband and children were very good, but they just couldn't understand why I was suddenly so difficult for eight or nine days. It is a very difficult thing to explain to people. You know you are feeling awful and ill and depressed but when you say it, it sounds rather silly. I made my family's life a misery at that time, and then felt terribly guilty, desperately trying to make amends the rest of the time.

'About a year after all this started, I began to get headaches too, nearly every month for the last two days before my period. Those were really the last straw. I got nervy and edgy and even more depressed and no amount of painkillers seemed to have a lasting effect. I used to go to my doctor but he just gave me tranquillisers and told me it was all part of being a woman. He was sympathetic, but he didn't really know what to do.'

In fact Stella's story has a happy ending. She went to a special clinic for PMT sufferers, was treated and is now back to her usual weight, and restored to good health and good humour.

'I feel completely different since getting treatment. It is hard to explain, but I feel as if I am myself now all month long. My pre menstrual headaches have completely gone and, though I still put on a little weight before my period, it is nothing to what used to happen. Best of all, I no longer get the terrible depressions. My husband and children have all remarked on the change in me. I have started working part-time – I feel confident enough to do that now. It is as if I have shed five years of being someone else and have become the same woman I was before I suffered from PMT.'

Chapter Three

What causes Pre Menstrual Tension?

'Why do I suffer such miseries before my period, doctor?
    What's the matter with me?'
'It's because you are a woman, my dear.'
'What can I do about it?'
'Nothing, you'll have to learn to live with it, I'm afraid.'

For years that sort of conversation went on in doctors
surgeries, and sometimes still does. Little research was done

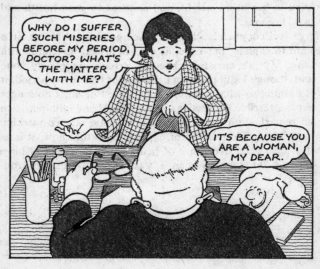

to try to understand why some women suffer so badly around the time of their periods.

Some doctors believed that, just as childbirth can be painful, so the menstrual cycle which prepared for that can be painful too. Unfortunate for the sufferers perhaps, but just something they would have to learn to live with. Or it was assumed that some women complain more than others, and have a lower tolerance of pain. And that other women are just 'neurotic' and imagine pains where none exist. Mostly the advice to them was pull themselves together and stop complaining.

Of course, some doctors felt differently. They were sympathetic and tried to find out whether something was actually wrong. Could it be, they wondered, that there was a physical cause? That in some women the menstrual cycle simply worked less efficiently than in others? Over the last 30 or 40 years, a handful of doctors in the United Kingdom, Europe and the United States have searched for answers.

One problem they were up against was that the menstrual cycle is one of the most complicated bodily functions.

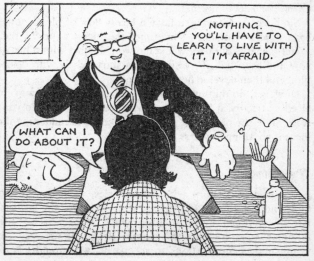

It was very difficult to find out exactly what was happening when. But modern methods of research and analysis have helped considerably and doctors have now been able to unravel some, though by no means all, of what occurs.

What is the menstrual cycle?

The term 'menstruation' probably makes you think of monthly bleeding. But it also covers what is going on before and after bleeding occurs.

Menstruation begins at puberty, anywhere between the age of ten and sixteen. It is the main sign that you are no longer a little girl but are rapidly growing into a woman. Your hips broaden, your breasts swell, you start growing pubic hair and profound chemical or hormonal changes in your body lead to emotional changes.

Menstruation varies from woman to woman. We generally think of the menstrual cycle as lasting 28 days, but that is only an average figure. Some women menstruate every 21 days, others go for as long as 36 days between periods, but all are considered normal.

Similarly, some women have a heavy flow of blood, some have a very light flow, sometimes the blood is bright red, sometimes it is dark brown, some women start with a heavy flow and then tail off, while others start lightly with 'spotting' and then develop heavier bleeding.

However, no matter how long your cycle is, or how your bleeding occurs, it is the same basic process at work in you. It is only if the pattern of your period changes suddenly that there is anything to worry about.

What happens?

Every woman is born with two ovaries, each containing thousands of unripe egg cells. After puberty, the ovaries release one egg every month, which travels down the fallopian tube towards the womb. Before it arrives, the womb makes preparations to receive it, with hundreds of tiny changes taking place in its walls.

44

As the egg travels towards the womb, two things are possible.

1. If you have had intercourse, then a sperm from the man may have made its way up through your vagina, through your womb and into the fallopian tube and fertilised the egg. In that case, the fertilised egg will travel down into the womb and attach itself to the womb's lining, where it will be nourished as it develops into a foetus.

2. If you have not had intercourse, the egg will enter your womb unfertilised. Even if you have had intercourse, there is a good chance that the egg will still not meet up with a sperm. In either case, the egg will cling to the lining for a few days and then the lining and egg together are washed out of your body – your period.

That is the egg cell's journey at its simplest. The complicated questions, to which we can give only some of the answers, are exactly how this process is begun and carried through. How do all the various parts of the body know **how** to act and **when** to act?

The hypothalamus is the control centre of the menstrual cycle. It is situated in the lower part of the brain and is about the size of a walnut.

The pituitary gland sits just below the hypothalamus and is linked to it by various pathways. The pituitary gland is the junior partner of the control centre.

The hormones are chemical agents sent out by the glands of the body. The hypothalamus and pituitary are particularly important as they control the activity of a number of other glands such as the ovaries, (testes in men) and adrenals. The hormones travel along your blood stream. When they arrive at the part of your body to which they have been sent, they cause certain changes to occur. There are many different hormones, but the important ones for our story are oestrogen, progesterone and prolactin.

*　　*　　*

The process which ends in your period begins with the

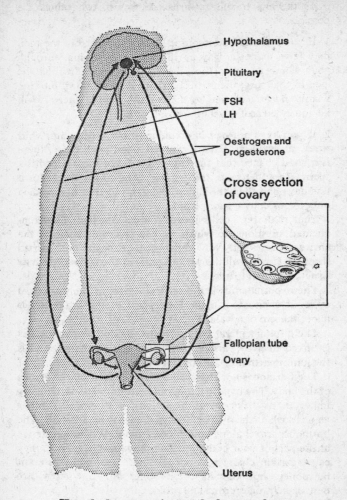

Hypothalamus

Pituitary

FSH
LH

Oestrogen and Progesterone

Cross section of ovary

Fallopian tube

Ovary

Uterus

How the hormones in your body control your period.
Cross section of ovary shows the release of the egg and the development of the corpus luteum.

hypothalamus. It stimulates the pituitary gland to produce a hormone which travels to the ovaries. There are waiting thousands of eggs, each with a tiny protective sac round itself, called a follicle. The hormone from the pituitary gland, called follicle stimulating hormone (FSH) does just that – it stimulates one of the follicles to start developing.

As the follicle develops, it produces a hormone called oestrogen, which travels to the womb. This makes the womb lining prepare for the egg's arrival.

After a few more days, the pituitary gland sends a second hormone to the ovaries. This is called the lutenising hormone (LH). Its job is to 'spring' the egg from the follicle. The follicle tears open and the egg begins its journey down the fallopian tubes towards the womb. This is ovulation.

As the egg travels onward, the scar it leaves behind changes into a yellow gland, the corpus luteum. This produces more of the hormone oestrogen and some of the hormone progesterone. The oestrogen rebuilds the womb lining after menstruation while progesterone stimulates the thickening of the womb lining preparing it to receive the fertilised egg. Please note that this has nothing to do with progestogen or any other of the ingredients usually found in the contraceptive pill.

The third hormone which is important in this process is called prolactin. Prolactin is secreted by the pituitary gland and affects the way FSH and LH influence the ovaries and the corpus luteum. What this means is that prolactin can alter the amounts of progesterone and oestrogen that are secreted during the cycle.

Hormone Imbalance

So what goes wrong to cause PMT? As I have said, there are no easy answers. But for some time doctors suspected that the problem lay in the amount of hormones, oestrogen and progesterone, which were being produced. Up to now, it has been very difficult to measure the amount of a particular hormone you have in your blood at any one time. But a new technique called radioimmunoassay has made this much easier, although it is still a difficult and expensive process and not yet widely used.

At St Thomas's Hospital in London, Professor Taylor and Dr Brush used radioimmunoassay in a study which has produced some very interesting results. They found that 40% or nearly half the women who suffered from PMT were **progesterone deficient.** This means that the level of progesterone in their bodies was not as high as it should be at the critical point in the menstrual cycle, when progesterone is supposed to be at its peak to stimulate the thickening of the womb lining.

At the same time, they found that 40% of the women had more **oestrogen** in their blood than expected. Some of these women had normal levels of progesterone, but because they had too much oestrogen, the **balance** between the levels of the two hormones was upset. It seems you need the right balance between the two just as you need the right balance between flour and fat to make a successful cake.

What is more, some of these women were also progesterone deficient, which meant that not only did they have too much oestrogen, they had too little progesterone as

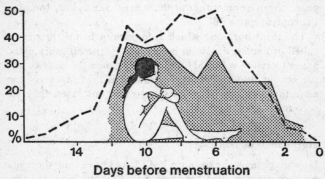

Days before menstruation

Comparison between the level of progesterone in a normal woman and in a woman suffering from PMT.
(Broken line indicates normal level of progesterone.
Unbroken line indicates level of progesterone in a woman suffering from PMT.)

well. Of course, this made the imbalance between the two hormones even worse.

Professor Taylor and Dr Brush concluded from this that a large number of women who suffer from PMT either have too little progesterone in their bodies at a crucial time, or they have too much oestrogen in relation to progesterone. Other things contribute to the belief that an imbalance between these two hormones is one of the main causes of PMT. For a start, PMT only occurs on those days of the cycle when progesterone should be present, and at a relatively high level. After menstruation, for instance, when progesterone disappears naturally anyway, the symptoms of PMT never occur.

Similarly, women who suffer most severely from PMT usually find that it disappears miraculously while they are pregnant, a time when the placenta is producing extra progesterone to nourish the growing baby.

Many women, too, find that their PMT problems only start after the birth of their first child. This is because once the baby is born, the extra supplies of progesterone and oestrogen that were nourishing it are shut off. Normal functioning should then resume, but sometimes it does not. Your hormones never settle down to their regular flow again and so imbalance develops, causing PMT.

There may also be an added explanation. St Thomas's Hospital found that a small number of women, 5%, who suffered from PMT, had **too much prolactin** in their blood, and that many more women had 'high normal' levels of prolactin, which means that they were close to the borderline between the right amount of prolactin and too much. Extra prolactin in the blood can upset the mechanisms controlling the production of oestrogen and progesterone by the ovaries. And this in turn can upset you. Prolactin also has other effects on the glands in the reproductive system and in the breasts.

Exactly why these imbalances occur has not been established for sure. Some doctors have suggested that it is a hereditary phenomenon, passed from mother to daughter. Others even argue that it simply goes to prove that modern women, finally released from the constant cycle of child bearing and suckling, are having difficulty because they now menstruate 'more than their bodies can stand'!

Investigations into the delicate and easily-disturbed hormonal balance is going on all the time. The fact is nevertheless that the basic root origin – or aetiology, as it is termed medically – is unknown. This is neither new or unusual. There are many other medical conditions which are well known and described: doctors know exactly what happens, but they still cannot say why.

The Hypothalamus and Pituitary Gland

This still leaves some women who do not appear to have any obvious hormone imbalance at all and yet suffer from PMT. This means that something else must be involved as well, and brings us back to the hypothalamus and pituitary gland.

You will remember that together they form the control centre for the menstrual cycle. They are also two of the most complicated and least understood parts of the body. They are linked to each other in a number of different ways and have a very delicate inter-relationship which doctors do not fully understand yet.

But we do know that various substances must be present for their relationship to function effectively. One of these essential substances is pyridoxine (also known as Vitamin B6).

Certain amounts of pyridoxine must be present in sufficient quantities before certain processes, like the proper production of oestrogen and progesterone, can take place.

Some women have below average levels of pyridoxine, it is believed. This lack, it seems, can have a harmful effect on the hypothalamus and on the two pathways, and upset your periods.

Why do the symptoms develop?

After reading Chapters One and Two, or if you suffer from PMT, you will know how many symptoms there are. It is still not clear why all of these develop, but we do know the reason why at least some of them occur.

We know, for instance, that oestrogen and progesterone can influence the amount of fluid present in your body at any one time. So if there is an imbalance in the levels of these two hormones, it is quite likely that water retention and bloatedness will result.

The hormone called prolactin is known to affect your breasts, and in the St Thomas's studies, the women who had too much, or 'high normal' levels of prolactin, almost always had very tender, swollen, and enlarged breasts in the days before their period.

The hypothalamus is important, too, because it not only controls the menstrual cycle, it also controls a variety of other things like appetite, weight, water balance and even your moods. Any or all of these may be disturbed during PMT, and any disturbance of the normal functioning of the hypothalamus could obviously be the reason. In particular, this might help to explain why mood swings are so common with PMT, when you feel irritable and depressed by turns, especially as the levels of progesterone and oestrogen present in your body can also have an effect on mood.

*   *   *

The psychological causes of PMT

So far in this chapter I have only talked about the physical causes of PMT. They are the key to understanding PMT and their discovery has meant that good, effective treatments have been found to help the millions of women who suffer.

But there are psychological causes of PMT, too, and they should not be ignored.

As you probably already know, your body is very sensitive to changes in your mood and state of mind. One of the most obvious examples of this is the reaction to fear. Fear is a psychological reaction to something that is happening to you or around you, and it can start a chain of reactions in your body. Your heart beats faster, you sweat, your hair stands on end, blood drains from your face as it rushes to your vital organs and adrenalin is pumped through your body to help you run fast, fight better and so on. In extreme cases of fear, your hair can turn grey overnight.

Tension and anxiety can also cause illnesses, like stomach ulcers for instance, and doctors are still trying to work out the connection between stress and heart attacks, strokes and the like. Some people notice that they get spots or dandruff when they are under pressure.

It is well known that stress and anxiety can alter the timing of your periods so that they become irregular or stop altogether. Similarly, stress and anxiety can affect you before your period and bring on PMT.

Stress and anxiety can be caused by circumstances, or your personality, or a mixture of both. If you are highly strung and a worrier, your level of tension is high anyway. This does not mean that you will necessarily suffer from PMT but it might make it more likely that you will. Your high level of anxiety might be enough to disrupt the smooth flow of hormones in your body and cause some of your symptoms. Or it might make relatively minor, mild symptoms worse. And your symptoms are more likely to be the psychological ones than the physical ones.

A naturally robust, calm woman might find her sore breasts a nuisance, and feel a bit lower than usual with PMT. But if you are highly strung you might find the same discomfort intolerable and your 'low' might sink to rock bottom.

Difficult circumstances can also put pressure on you which can affect your menstrual cycle. A divorce, the death of someone you love, or simply a pile up of problems at home and work may make you feel strained and anxious enough to bring on PMT. It is not always easy to tell how far such psychological pressures are responsible, but occasionally you come across women whose personality or circumstances make it easier to say: 'her PMT is obviously partly caused by psychological factors' or 'her PMT is obviously caused only by physical factors'. Two such women are Mary and Jane.

Mary is 28 years old with three children, one of whom, Simon, has recurrent physical illness and is slightly mentally retarded as well. He has always been a great worry to her, and the occasion of numerous rows with her husband, Bill. They live in a small flat, which does not really have sufficient space for the family, especially Simon, but they cannot afford to move. Money is another worry.

So Mary's circumstances are difficult. But she is also the first to admit that she is 'nervy'. 'I was a nervous child, very shy and withdrawn. And I am a bit of a worrier, I know, and having Simon has not helped. People have suggested putting him in a home. We did try once, but I'm glad they could not take him because I felt awful about sending him away. He might be a handful sometimes, but he is my son and I love him.'

It seems very likely that the combination of Mary's personality and her circumstances contribute a great deal to her PMT, although the underlying cause is physical. It is no surprise that she suffers mostly psychological symptoms, particularly tension and depression.

Jane, on the other hand, is a cheerful, calm woman. She is 31, married with two children, a girl and a boy. They are not wealthy, but they are comfortably off and have a pleasant house. Jane is the sort of woman who takes things in her stride. 'I always say, "what's the use of worrying, it never was worthwhile" – to quote the old song. Well, it never is, is it?'

Jane gets several physical symptoms of PMT. She puts on weight and gets bad headaches. But she also finds that she is much quicker tempered during the three or four days before her period. 'That used to bother me terribly until Mike, my husband, noticed the connection with my period. I thought there was something the matter with me, mentally. It all started after my son was born. I would suddenly get into a terrible rage and give him a good whack if he so much as looked at me. You wouldn't believe it, but I am really against hitting children, for anything. That's why I couldn't understand what had come over me.'

There is such a clear difference between Jane's personality most of the time and her personality in the days before her periods, that it is obvious that it is physical, not psychological causes that underly her PMT. But some women are not so easy to diagnose, and a mixture of the two may be at the bottom of their PMT.

It is sometimes very hard to separate the psychological **causes** from the psychological **symptoms** of PMT. For example, your irritability and depression (psychological symptoms) may be caused by the physical imbalance in your hormones. Or your anxiety, or a tendency to depression (psychological causes) or even particularly stressful circumstances leading to anxiety may all be important factors in bringing on PMT. It is not always clear which came first, nor how one affects the other. You can, in fact, find yourself on a very unpleasant downward spiral. Your hormone control mechanism is upset so that you get PMT. This produces the physical and psychological symptoms we have discussed and makes you feel much worse, which means that you are more stressed generally, not just before your period. But this, of course, can make your PMT worse, too, and so on in a miserable spiral.

It is important, however, to understand that psychological factors are never all that is involved in PMT. They may be one cause of your PMT. They may be your worst symptoms. But the root cause of PMT, no matter how it was originally triggered, is physical, and can be treated. Of course, this will not miraculously cause all your problems to disappear. If you are tense anyway, you are not suddenly going to change. If your life is full of stresses, these will not suddenly resolve themselves. Mary, for example, has been having treatment for PMT for some months now. She is much better than she was, but she still gets tense and depressed sometimes, particularly just before her period. Unless her circumstances or personality change, it is likely that she will always have some problems.

Treating PMT can help to reduce or even get rid of the physical and psychological symptoms and this can relieve you of at least one extra burden. You no longer have to fear the week or so before your period and this, in turn, may make some of your other problems seem a little less of a burden.

*   *   *

It is worth mentioning here that **period pains** are not the same thing as PMT.

Very few women escape period pains of some sort at some stage of their life but you should not assume that all period pains are a part of PMT. There are in fact two sorts of period pain, one associated with PMT and one not, and since they both have different causes, it is important not to muddle the two.

Congestive dysmenorrhoea

Dysmenorrhoea is simply the medical term for period pains, so do not let it confuse you. Some doctors refer to one type of dysmenorrhoea as congestive dysmenorrhoea, which is a rather vague term for what is essentially PMT. We have already described the symptoms in detail in Chapter One: bloatedness, a dull ache in the stomach, possibly backache and headaches are some of the most obviously painful symptoms. The important thing is that these all occur in the week, or sometimes even ten days, before your period is due and disappear as soon as your period has started.

Spasmodic dysmenorrhoea

Spasmodic dysmenorrhoea starts where PMT ends, although it is not common for one woman to suffer from both, which is some consolation! You get spasms of dull or acute pain in the lower abdomen and genital area when your period starts, sometimes accompanied by a heavy, dragging feeling, and pains in the top and inside of your thighs and the lower part of your back. These period pains normally only last for two or three days and disappear when your period starts to fade.

The spasmodic cramps you feel may be caused by the actions of the muscles of your womb, as they slough off the lining that was prepared in case an egg was fertilised and needed nourishing. It is possible, too, that these muscles have not received sufficient oestrogen to mature them and they have difficulty stretching. Or the neck of the womb may be small and pressure on it as the blood forces its way through causes painful stretching. Usually these sort of period pains only last during your teens or early twenties and rarely recur after the birth of a baby, which of course stretches the muscles of the womb lining and the neck of the womb.

Sometimes, they can be quite mild, but for some women the pain and cramping can be very severe to the point when they are actually sick and have to retreat to bed with a hot water bottle until the pains subside.

Recently, doctors in America and Britain have found that new drugs called anti-prostaglandins have helped a great many women with severe menstrual cramps. You may like to ask your doctor about this. I look in detail at treatments specifically for PMT in Chapter Eleven.

The two types of dysmenorrhoea need to be carefully distinguished so that the correct treatment can be given. Obviously, if you mistake one for the other and treat it accordingly, you will simply make it worse.

Chapter Four

Blood Secrets

What were your feelings about your period when you first started menstruating? Were you embarrassed at the very idea of menstruation? Did you find it hard to discuss with girlfriends, or with your parents? What is your attitude now? Do you still find it hard to talk about menstruation? Do you blush when the word is mentioned? Do you think of your periods as a messy necessity to be tolerated each month?

If you answered 'yes' to many of these questions, you are not alone. A great many women feel anxious or embarrassed about their periods. Sometimes this attitude starts very early. Perhaps you were made to feel worried about your periods when you were younger, as if they were something dirty or shameful, and so you came to dread them. Or, if you knew nothing about them, you may have been very frightened when you first started bleeding. Or your attitude may have developed as you got older and saw that other people were embarrassed when menstruation was mentioned.

Some people believe that your attitude to your periods can affect the way you experience them. If you are anxious about them now or if, unconsciously, old anxieties from your childhood linger on, these feelings may add a stress as your period approaches. And this stress may contribute to your PMT.

Of course, you are not bound to suffer from PMT just

because you do not particularly like your periods. And many women who do suffer from PMT have never felt any anxiety about their periods. But it is worth exploring how your attitude to your period was formed in case this is a contributory cause of your PMT. And I think it is a good idea to uncover some of the reasons why, even today, when we are all much franker and more outspoken, so many men and women still find menstruation difficult to discuss.

* * *

Your attitude to your period develops not simply as a result of what you think but also through the way society views menstruation, how you were introduced to menstruation by your parents or teachers and their attitude to it, and how your friends reacted when you first started menstruating. Obviously all these things will play a greater or lesser part in forming your attitude to menstruation, depending on how strong an influence they had or have on you. But none of us can completely escape from the pressure of ideas that are generally held however much we may disagree with them.

Society's attitude

When you think of all the nasty names attached to menstruation – 'the curse', 'the blues', 'feeling indisposed' to name but a few – it is almost a surprise that any of us come through thinking that there is a **positive** side to menstruation! Society, since way back when, has generally treated menstruation as something to be ashamed of and hidden away, in contrast to pregnancy (the other side of menstruation) which is a proud event to be announced and welcomed. In many early primitive societies, women were, and in some tribes still are, banished from the main house and made to stay in a private hut during menstruation. They may not bathe, eat or touch their bodies, and have to remain in a crouched position the whole time. Above all, no men can come near them during this time, for fear of their lives.

In other societies, women have to drink and eat with

separate utensils and must not prepare food for men for fear that men will be contaminated and become diseased or, worse still, die. At different times and in different cultures menstruating women have been held responsible for blighting crops, turning wine to vinegar or copper green, causing mirrors to dull, sharp metal to blunt, causing mares or cows to miscarry and killing anything from pests to bees, horses or cattle.

What underlies a lot of this is the belief that the menstruating woman is possessed by an evil spirit that lives in her blood, and can exert a power to harm. For some, the monthly flow of blood is the curse that God laid upon Eve, and hence all women, because she led Adam into sin. Even today, though we may think that we are emancipated from some of these beliefs, they live on and pop up in unexpected places. Not long ago there was a reference to the 'curse of Eve' in a popular American television comedy series called 'All in the Family'. Archie Bunker, the main character, reflected a popular view in society when he said 'Read your Bible. Read about Adam and Eve . . . Going against direct orders, she makes poor Adam take a bite out of that apple. So God got sore and told them to get their clothes on and get outta there. So it was Eve's fault God cursed women with this trouble. That's why they call it, what do you call it, the curse.'

Several religions impose a variety of rules to be observed during menstruation. At the beginning of this century, Greek Orthodox women were forbidden to take communion while menstruating. Manu Hindu law decrees: 'A woman during her menstrual period shall retire for three days to a place apart. During this time she shall not look at anybody not even her own children or at the light of the sun. On the fourth day she shall bathe.'

Orthodox Judaism forbids sexual activity during menstruation. At the end of the period, a woman must go to the mikvah, a ritual bath, and be cleansed. Only after the mikvah can she have sexual relations again. The Catholic Church, too, used to urge abstinence during a period. The assumption was that a woman is unclean at this time and so should not be touched, which reinforces the feeling that there is something not quite 'nice' about menstruation. In fact, many non-religious women prefer to avoid sexual intercourse during their periods. They do not think this is because they are avoiding contamination by an evil spirit nor because they are observing a religious taboo. They feel that while they are bleeding, intercourse is messy. It is hard to know how far this dirty feeling is part of a general sense that society thinks of menstruation as dirty.

Looking round, you can see how far society pushes menstruation to the back of its mind, out of the way where it cannot easily intrude. Until fairly recently there were very few advertisements for sanitary products and even now those there are tend to show everything except the sanitary towel, or tampon, itself. Many women are still embarrassed when buying sanitary towels and I am sure very few stop to ask the shop assistant for advice on which is the best. This is something that often even friends find hard to discuss.

It is also interesting to try to find the words for sanitary towel or tampon in a foreign phrase book. The chances are you will not, even though the words for buying a sanitary towel might be much more useful than a lot of other words or phrases that you will find. Somehow periods and their paraphernalia are 'women's business' to be dealt with discreetly on their own without involving or embarrassing the men.

I've often thought that shaving for men is an interesting comparison. I know it is not as bloody as menstruation (well, not usually anyway!) but it is certainly messy and not something that I would want to do every day. And, like menstruation for women, it is a sign in men that they have reached puberty. Imagine how ridiculous it would seem if men were embarrassed to mention shaving and felt ashamed as their 'five o'clock shadow' appeared every day. After all, it is part of being a man.

It is not an exact analogy of course, but it is worth thinking about: after all, menstruation is part of being a woman.

Your parent's attitude

It is very hard to know how much you are affected by the way in which your parents introduced you to your period and their general attitude to it. Very little research has been done to find out about this, so a lot of what I am saying is tentative and based on clinical observation by a variety of doctors and psychologists and conversations with women themselves. There does seem to be a tendency for girls who have had little or no explanation about their periods beforehand, or whose parents were obviously very embarrassed to talk about periods, to feel apprehension around the time of their period even many years after they first started menstruating.

Some parents and in particular mothers, who are traditionally supposed to be the ones to prepare their daughters for menstruation, find it very difficult to talk about menstruation at all. They change the subject whenever it is brought up or give short, embarrassed answers that often leave their daughters more confused than ever. This embarrassment is also, of course, very quickly conveyed to the child. I spoke to many women who remembered that when they were children they soon found out that 'where did baby brother come from?' and 'what is a period?' were two questions that never got a straight answer. The association of menstruation with the difficult subject of 'sex' is very natural of course, since it is all part of the reproductive cycle, but that adds yet another reason why menstruation is difficult to discuss.

Some mothers, to cover their embarrassment, go into very elaborate and detailed scientific explanations that do not seem to relate to your body at all. Anthea, who suffers from quite severe PMT now, recognises that she has been anxious about her periods since she was a very little girl.

'I remember when I was about ten that I had heard that there was something called "a period" but no one seemed very clear what it was. My mother sat me down and gave me a long explanation with drawings which I could not follow at all. I think mostly she talked about rabbits and baby rabbits and I never really saw the connection. She never once mentioned that I would bleed.

'When my period did happen I thought something awful was wrong with me, especially because I could not work out what the brownish stain in my pants was. My best friend said that I had probably eaten a sticky sweet the night before and it had come out the other end. I did not eat sweets for ages after that but it soon became clear that the leak continued no matter what I ate.'

It is surprising how often explanations about the reproductive cycle leave out the fact that you are going to bleed quite heavily for a few days each month. As a result, a lot of women thought they had cancer or a terrible wasting disease. I myself was quite well up on 'reproduction' and 'how babies are made' by the time my period came and yet I can still remember the shock of seeing so much blood flowing out of me. No one had remembered to prepare me for that. And certainly the mysteries of sanitary towels, belts and pins were quite unexpected and hard to cope with when I was still trying to sort out what the bleeding actually meant.

Even model parents who try to be frank cannot always quite overcome embarrassment, or escape society's attitude that periods and menstruation are something to be talked about secretly, in private. When asked about it in the middle of a public gathering, which quite often happens, they hastily say 'I'll tell you later' and do, when they are far away from other ears.

Women who are themselves embarrassed about their periods or suffer from PMT are likely to pass this anxiety on to their daughters. I would not be surprised if further research showed that PMT runs in families. Not only is there a likelihood that there is an inherited tendency to suffer, but daughters may well see their mothers' miseries and expect the same. Your expectation of what your period is going to be like can affect the way that you experience it too. If you fear the worst, then you may unconsciously look for symptoms or become tense and nervous as you expect them to appear. And, of course, these tensions can increase your chance of suffering from PMT.

If you were brought up in a strictly religious background this can make a difference too, in part because of the rituals we spoke of earlier. There is a tradition in the Jewish religion, for example, that young girls are slapped on the face the day they start menstruating to bring the blood to their cheeks as it flows from their vagina. Many Jewish women whose mothers slapped them had no idea why and often found it rather frightening.

'I thought I had done something wrong and, although my mother quickly explained that the slap was not a punishment but a tradition, I sometimes still get the feeling that I am being naughty when I get my period.'

One Irish girl, Marie, who was brought up in a strict Catholic family, remembers her first period very clearly.

'One day I started to bleed unexpectedly from my vagina. I rushed to my mother and asked her what had happened, thinking that I had caught some terrible disease. She looked panic stricken, nervously told me to be quiet and come to the bathroom at once and there, with the door tightly shut, she explained that all women bleed once a month but that I was not to mention this to anyone, especially not my father, and I was to be sure the blood did not go over everywhere.'

Marie suffers from bad PMT and, thinking about it now, feels sure that some at least of her problems are due to the years she spent hiding all the evidence of her periods from her family. Some research in America backs this up. It was found that women from strongly religious backgrounds, particularly Jewish and Catholic, where the menstrual taboos were known about or practised, were more likely to suffer from PMT.

It is not hard to understand, too, why parents from all backgrounds often have mixed feelings about their daughters' puberty. On the one hand it is a good and positive thing because it means that she is becoming a full woman, fertile, normal and able to have babies. But on the other hand it presents the problems of developing sexuality, of boyfriends, virginity and pregnancy. Worries about how they and their daughter are going to cope with her newfound womanhood can make even the most enthusiastic parents hesitate as they say 'congratulations, today you are a woman'.

The attitude of your friends

School children can be very cruel to each other, sometimes without meaning to be. Many women remember to this day the attitude of their friends when they first started menstruating.

'I started menstruating when I was very young, just after 10, and though I did everything I could to hide it, somehow everyone in my class seemed to know. Everywhere I went there seemed to be people nudging each other and giggling. I thought I was a freak.'

The one thing, it seems, that many people forget to tell their children is **when** menstruation is likely to occur. The 'normal' age range is very wide – anything from 11–16 – yet many women who started menstruating well within that range thought they were abnormal. In fact the age you start menstruating can make all the difference. If you started before most of your friends, they may have been very suspicious of you and taken their resentment and jealousy that you 'got there first' out on you by teasing, which in turn could make you feel very embarrassed and shy. At that age it is often hard to be different.

On the other hand, if you started your period after most of your friends, that could be even worse. You feel tense and anxious, sure that there is something wrong with you, and your friends rub it in, enjoying knowing something you don't. They are mature women now, they imply, you are still a little girl. There is some truth in that, of course. The menarche, as the start of menstruation is called, is an important time because it marks the start of a cyclical rhythm of the sex hormones which underlies not only fertility, but also biological and emotional changes which will continue for the next 40 years. The feelings and ideas of a girl who starts her period whether earlier or later than her contemporaries, can affect a young woman's idea of herself, how 'grown up' she feels, how sexy, how attractive to boys and her evaluation of her worth in relation to her friends, both girls and boys.

All that I have said so far may have made the onset of your period seem only an unpleasant and upsetting experience. Of course, for many women the start of their period is a joyful event. They swop experiences with friends, they become women together, and they enjoy feeling mature and watching the development of their breasts and pubic hair. For them, the joys far outweigh their apprehensions. And yet, as I said at the beginning, some of these women may develop PMT.

Similarly, by no means all the women who have had bad memories of the onset of their periods **will** develop PMT. We simply do not know how far your attitude to your period affects your experience of it, and we do know that there are **physical** reasons for PMT to develop. How the two inter-relate still needs unravelling. But it does seem ridiculous that, in an age when we are so much franker and more explicit about sex, so many women still find it difficult to talk openly about and feel at ease with their periods. Even if our attitudes are too deeply set to change, let's hope that we can try to avoid instilling fear and shame into our children. Perhaps that way, gradually, society's attitude too will change.

Chapter Five

Women and Men

PMT does not just affect you, it affects all the people you come into contact with. At work you may be less cheerful than usual, or sharper tongued without people taking too much notice. But it is at home, where you are less likely to restrain your behaviour, that the effect on those around you can be worst.

Your guard drops, and feelings that you had bottled up erupt unexpectedly. You snap at your husband or children without apparent reason, ready to pick a fight over anything. Lois, who has two small children, was just like that.

'My husband, Jack, could see the signs that I was getting into my "moody patch" as he called it, so he would think "I must be especially nice to Lois today" and he would come home with a little present for me. Of course, I'd lose my temper: "What do you want to go wasting money on presents for? You know we can't afford it. Haven't you got anything better to do with your money", that sort of thing. So the next month he would decide not to bring me a present but just be gentle and loving. Well, I would fly into a rage again. "Why haven't you brought me a present? You don't really love me, you never bring me presents" and nothing he said would appease me. He led an impossible life, and I felt terribly guilty during the good times in between. Thank goodness I managed to get treatment!'

Sometimes your husband or boyfriend may be the first to

notice a pattern in your behaviour, seeing it long before you do, even though he cannot always put a name to it. It may be that the change in your personality each month coincides with some activity he does regularly, or it may be simply that he realises that you are not like that **all** the time and together you work out the connection with your periods.

Professor Taylor who ran a pre menstrual clinic at St Thomas's Hospital in London for three years, found that PMT was the complaint which most often involved husbands as well as their wives. The husbands insisted on coming along too, to give their wives moral support and to make sure that their wives told the doctor everything!

Of course, PMT is not the only thing that causes problems between you and your husband or boyfriend. But it does make a difference. It can mean that small arguments develop into full-scale rows, when you say things you regret later. Or you might not be as responsive as usual to your husband's or boyfriend's needs and brush him aside when he wants your help.

Sometimes it can have totally unexpected effects. Dr Dalton tells the story of a salesman whose commission dropped severely once a month, putting a financial strain on the family and worrying the salesman a great deal. Dr Dalton charted his wife's menstrual cycle and found that she suffered from severe PMT. This affected her husband, who became anxious and distracted and so less efficient at his job. The drop in his commission coincided with her pre menstrual days. Dr Dalton treated his wife and cured the salesman!

When the problem goes unrecognised for a long time, the strains on your marriage can be immense, even if your husband is understanding. In the end there is often not much he can do to help, and you just have to let your moodiness take its course. If neither of you realises that there is a pattern, then you seem a bad-tempered or 'neurotic' woman to him, and you probably secretly worry about yourself too sometimes. As Mary, who is now 46 and beginning to face the menopause, put it:

'It never occurred to me or my husband that my totally

unreasonable behaviour towards my husband and family over the years could have been caused by anything but basic viciousness in me.'

Her husband put up with her moods as best he could, and the children kept well out of reach. But Mary's suffering often made all their lives miserable, and until recently they never knew the reason why.

You may find, as many women do, that as far as your husband, boyfriend or the family goes, irritability is your most upsetting symptom. Usually you may be able to curb your temper and lash out with your tongue, not your fists. But you may sometimes find that aggression builds up inside you, you cannot control it and it explodes viciously and physically. Some women throw plates, vases, knives or anything that is to hand at the time. Others punch, kick and maul their husbands.

Obviously, if this happens to you it is disturbing for your husband, but it can also be very frightening for you too. You feel out of control and unable to stop. 'It is as if I am possessed' is how several women describe it or 'It is as if something snaps in my head.' One woman was more explicit:

'I see the carving knife glistening on the work surface in the kitchen and, before I really stop to think, I've grabbed it and hurled it at my husband. Luckily, I'm not a very good shot and he is good at ducking, but I'm so afraid that one of these days I shall do him a terrible injury.'

Dr Dalton in her book 'Once a Month' quotes Roger Langley and Richard Levy, two researchers in Washington who have estimated that about 20% of all husbands in the United States (that is about 12 million men) are battered husbands, who suffer regular physical violence at the hands of their wives. They call it 'the most unreported crime'. It seems very likely that much of the 'crime' lies not in any basic viciousness in women but in the hormone imbalance they experience each month. I would not be surprised if further research showed that a disproportionate amount of husband battering occurred in the pre menstrual week, correlating with research already carried out on accidents, hospital admissions and crime. PMT does not cause the problem but it can contribute.

The other side of the question is what your husband does if you lash out at him like this. You may be lucky and have a gentle, tolerant husband who avoids you when you are in this mood and leaves the house at the first signs of violence. But, understandably perhaps, your husband may not be able to cope with your temper and hits back, sometimes himself becoming extremely violent. As you are probably physically the weaker of the two, you may suffer much more from his violence than he does from yours. Sonia, a 38 year old housewife, found that out the hard way:

'When I experience the depression, self pity, persecution and violent temper, it has repercussions on my husband, as he is unable to cope and becomes extremely violent in turn. On one or two occasions I have had to go to hospital afterwards.'

This throws a new light on a better-known problem than battered husbands – battered wives. There is no question that many women suffer dreadful, frightening violence from their husbands which they have done nothing at all to provoke. The reasons for this are very complicated and I cannot go into them here, but there are some obvious reasons why a man might hit his wife – if he is drunk, for instance, or under pressure at work, or in debt, or has a plain nasty temper.

A less obvious but important reason for this might be that his wife provokes him by her own violent behaviour when suffering from PMT. Of course this does not excuse his violence. A calmer, gentler man would walk away or keep his temper in check. But it does mean that the woman is likely to suffer violence again and again without understanding why, when there is a clear explanation and effective treatment.

If PMT is not recognised as one possible cause of this sort of violence, it is quite likely that the woman will get into trouble again. She may leave her husband, divorce and remarry and the man she chooses may have a similar personality to her first husband, because those are the sort of men she fancies. Her PMT provokes him and she is back to square one again. If her PMT had been recognised and treated they might have lived happily ever after.

* * *

As if your relationships were not under sufficient strain, your sex life when you are suffering from PMT can be disrupted as well. You may simply not feel like having sexual intercourse when you are so tense, irritable and depressed. And often your husband or boyfriend is not particularly keen either when you are in such an unpleasant mood.

But the sexual difficulties can be more complicated than that. You may feel very aroused at this time of the month and keen to make love but your tension makes it hard for you to show affection. Sarah was very explicit about this:

'I sometimes think I should be in a loony bin. I seem to

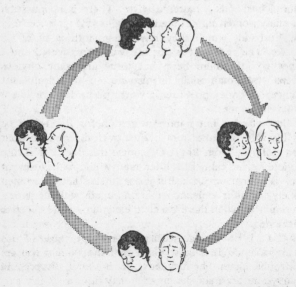

The vicious circle

really need and want my husband to cuddle me or love me in a special way when I am due on, but in some way I spoil it and push him away from me by causing an argument or picking on him for something silly.'

Giving or receiving affection can be very difficult when you are distressed, but your lack of responsiveness may be very hurtful to your husband or boyfriend. He feels rejected this time and so he may be reluctant to try another approach later in the week or month for fear he will be rejected again. By that time, of course, you may be feeling right as rain but he may not realise that or, by that time, he may not want to recognise it.

One of the most upsetting aspects of PMT is the effect it can have on your life **outside** the actual days of suffering. You feel better once your period arrives. But your husband is still feeling bitter and sore at your bad temper, moodiness and unresponsiveness. So, while you feel guilty and you try hard to make amends, he carries on sulking, or feels wary that this sudden cheerfulness on your part is only the prelude to yet another change of mood.

He may be unhelpful and cold towards you, and this makes you miserable or angry again, this time not because of your PMT but because of your husband's behaviour to you. The irony (which will be lost on both of you) is that PMT is at the bottom of it all, but now one step removed. This makes it even harder to detect because it seems as if you are depressed and irritable all the time.

With all the difficulties I have been describing, it would hardly be surprising if many marriages cracked under the strain. In fact, nobody knows how many divorces or separations PMT has occasioned because no research has been done to find out, and in any case it is hard to isolate one reason why couples split up. But conversations with sufferers and their families, and letters from them, as well as talks I have had with several doctors, make it clear that PMT has had a profound effect on many relationships. Many couples realise with hindsight (or some even saw at the time) that PMT was the final pressure that broke them up.

Occasionally the woman herself feels unable to manage

71

her family any more, or feels terribly guilty at all the misery she is causing them. Linda, the mother of two young boys, finally gave up:

'I knew my awful behaviour was connected with my periods and I could not bear the long-suffering look on my husband's face, and the fear of my temper in my children's eyes. I've left them now, and though I feel guilty as hell at having walked out, I feel relieved to be on my own. I am now seeking treatment and very much hope that as a result my husband and I will get back together again.'

Sometimes the departure is not so rational, especially if, as often happens, it takes place during the pre menstrual week.

'I got so bad recently that I left my husband, but before doing so I ripped the curtains down for apparently very little reason.'

Sometimes it is the husband who gives up, more often than not because he does not understand what is happening to his wife and simply feels he made a terrible mistake and married an evil-tempered or depressive woman. Rosemary's marriage has ended in divorce.

'My marriage broke up because my husband saw me as abnormal and inadequate.'

She is struggling to bring up her three year old daughter, and is finding it increasingly difficult. Obviously her husband did not understand her problem and nor at the time did she. But even understanding husbands cannot always take the strain.

'For a number of years my wife has spent two weeks out of four in awful misery. That is really no life at all and it is getting worse. We desperately need help. I feel that if we can't get help soon our marriage is going to break up.'

In fact his wife is being treated for PMT at the moment and her 'awful misery' is fast disappearing.

CASE HISTORY: SUSAN

Susan and her husband Ron, are both civil servants living in London. Susan started to suffer from PMT shortly after her first period and it has become increasingly worse over the years. She has been married to Ron for sixteen years, and they have no children. As Susan puts it: 'We didn't think we could cope with children as well as me, so we decided to have two cats instead!'

Susan gets PMT regularly every month, though some months it is slightly better than others. For her, the worst problem is the violent, uncontrollable tempers she gets into.

'It comes on during the day sometimes and I think, I'll cook something very nice for dinner, and I'll be nice to Ron, and I'll fight it. But it doesn't matter. I'll cook the meal and I'll think I don't want it, I don't like it. I'll go up on my bed and I'll just shut myself away, and I won't speak to anyone. And then, of course, when Ron comes and says, "Do come and eat your nice dinner, now that you have prepared it all," I fly at him and attack him. I grab hold of him and tear his jacket, hit him, rip all the buttons off his coat, I've smashed his glasses a good few times, too.

'The awful thing is that, even while I'm doing all this I don't want it to be this way. I want to be left alone but I also don't want to be left alone; I want Ron to come and comfort me. It is very complicated. I know I should be good and I should just say, "It will all pass". But it never does pass. It is something that is wound up inside, you know, like a great spring. And as soon as anything triggers it off I'm away. It is very frightening. Like being possessed I suppose.'

Ron is, fortunately for Susan, a tolerant non-violent man, but sometimes even he can take no more.

'I rather dread when I know Susan is coming on because I know what is going to happen. Very often when I come home from work I find the door locked and shut, so I can't get in. I have to try to persuade her through the letterbox to let me in. Sometimes, when she really lays into me and hits me, I do hit back. I just do not know what else to do.'

Susan's great fear has always been that she would become dangerous, to Ron or herself.

'I never ever hit Ron with anything, only my hands. But I do really hit him, smack him, punch him on the head. Sometimes I wake up at night and think: I hate you, and

73

start thumping him on the back – there is no escape for him. I am really terrified that I will pick up a knife one day and kill Ron, or that I would do something silly myself, like go to the railway station and throw myself under a train if I get into a great enough state. Sometimes I've suggested to Ron that he divorce me, although I didn't want him to. I couldn't bear the thought of being left alone. But I feel that maybe it would be best if we didn't live together, and that he found happiness somewhere else.'

But Ron is resilient, because, as he says, he knows that for three weeks out of four Susan is the bright happy person he loves and wants to stay with.

In fact, Susan has been treated with much success: 'I can't tell you the difference treatment has made. I don't smash plates, I don't attack Ron any more, I don't feel that sort of deep down hatred I used to feel. Of course I still lose my temper occasionally, but it can happen at any time, not just before my periods, and it is normal temper now, not those blinding rages of PMT. It is marvellous to be me all the time, and in full control.

'I'm much, much happier in myself now, and naturally my relationship with Ron has benefited enormously. I think we both see the change treatment has brought as a liberation after so many years of my pre menstrual ups and downs.'

Chapter Six

You and Your Children

Your children, especially when they are very young, are probably more sensitive to your mood changes than anyone else. This makes them particularly vulnerable if you suffer badly from PMT. Any increase of tension or irritability in you and they are liable to feel personally responsible. And, of course, if you have a splitting headache and are feeling cross and depressed, then you are much more likely to shout at them.

Even at the best of times, children can be very hard work. But when you are feeling heavy and lethargic, the daily routine of dressing them, preparing breakfast, getting them off to school, having tea ready when they return, washing and ironing their things, tidying up after them, can seem too much to manage. You flop down, exasperated, and burst into tears. When your children come home they find you red-eyed and perhaps try to be especially good, fearful that your sadness is in some way their fault. More likely, they are full of beans and keen to play, but you have no patience. Everything they do gets on your nerves, and there is no harmony until they are finally safely tucked up in bed.

Often, the effects of your pre menstrual behaviour on your children are hard to detect, and rather unexpected. Not long ago, Dr Dalton researched children's admissions into hospitals and their attendance at their local doctor's surgery. In both cases it was found that a much higher than expected proportion of the children's mothers, about half, (49% and 54% respectively) were in their pre menstrual week or the first days of their period when they brought their children in.

There are a variety of possible reasons for this surprising result. As we have seen, when you are suffering from PMT, even ordinary chores seem difficult to manage. So, if your children fall ill, even if they have only got a cold, cough or runny nose, you may feel unable to cope yourself. Instead of just putting them to bed with a hot drink and a dose of cough mixture, you rush them round to the doctor.

Also **you** may be the cause of your children's injuries because you are clumsier and more absentminded. You might spill boiling water while making a pot of tea, or let them get near the stove and pull a pan over themselves, when normally you would have been more watchful and quickly intervened before an accident could occur. You can probably think of numerous occasions when only your

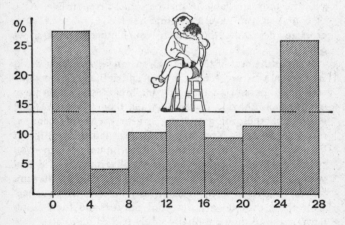

**Timing of children's surgery attendances and
mother's menstrual cycle.**
(Month is divided into four day periods starting with the
onset of menstruation. Dotted line indicates expected
incidence on a statistical basis.)

ability to 'get there first' prevented an accident. When you lose that ability temporarily, accidents can quickly multiply.

Some children, too, develop illnesses, problems like bed wetting for instance, brought on by emotional stress and upset rather than disease. Without realising it, there may be many ways in which your behaviour to your children can be disturbing for them while you are suffering from PMT.

Even if you know what the cause is, it is hard to tell your children that. As one mother put it: 'how do you explain to children that "mummy is peculiar" each month?' It is not simply that you lose your temper more quickly, though of course that can be bewildering for children if they cannot see that they have done anything wrong. You may also feel that you just do not want to be bothered with the children, and will not play with them, go for walks, or listen to their account of their day at school, all things that they generally expect.

Again, if your breasts are swollen and painful it is much harder to hug your children affectionately. They rush to you for a hug, and you wince. It may seem to your children that you are rejecting them, and because they cannot understand why, they feel unhappy and insecure. This in turn can make them ill, with coughs, colds or allergic reactions like asthma which may owe much more to their psychological unhappiness than to any physical problem. Treating the infection will not always eliminate the problem. The illness may well keep recurring or something else will develop.

Susan, a mother of a small boy, had just this problem. She used to take her son to play in a recreation ground near their home every afternoon. But after the birth of her second child, a little girl, she began to suffer from bad PMT. At the same time, her son started bed wetting. Initially her doctor thought it was because her son was jealous of his new sister and all the attention she was getting. But then she went to see Dr Dalton, who has a keen eye for PMT sufferers. She made Susan keep a chart of the dates when her PMT began and to record the days that her son wet his bed. His bed wetting coincided regularly with the week before his mother's period. In fact it turned out that Susan was so lethargic during those days that she did not bother to take her son to the park, and her breasts were so swollen and painful that she avoided hugging and cuddling him. Dr Dalton treated Susan's PMT and her son stopped bed wetting.

Some children, as they grow older, learn to spot the signs of their mothers' bad days and keep out of the way. One girl told me that she and her sister have a code to warn each other if Mum is on the warpath. Or sometimes fathers become conspiratorial with the children so that they all give mother a wide berth.

Dorothy, whose twin son and daughter are teenagers now, explained her PMT to them when they were eight years old.

'I didn't go into details, of course, but I just told them that it was something I went through each month and they should be prepared. I might seem cross or miserable but I didn't mean it really. They seemed to understand, at least they didn't get so anxious about my behaviour, and I think

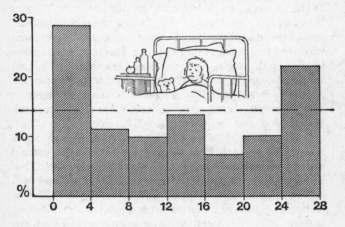

Timing of children's admissions to hospital and mother's menstrual cycle.
(Month is divided into four day periods starting with the onset of menstruation. Dotted line indicates expected incidence on a statistical basis.)

they really did try not to provoke me. And my husband talked it over too, so we sort of shared it as a family, which helped me.'

One of the benefits of your PMT, surprisingly, may be that your husband plays a more active part in looking after the children, especially if you both know what the matter is. He may well help bath the children, or change nappies, or if they are older, spend more time with them in the evenings when you are feeling particularly low or irritable. They may naturally turn to him anyway, for help with homework or for a game, if they know they are not likely to get a warm response from you.

Battered babies

As we saw in the last chapter, pre menstrual bad temper can sometimes go beyond verbal abuse to physical violence. It can make you violent, or it can provoke violence in your husband.

Sometimes, inevitably, the children also get involved. They may see the row between you and your husband and this could frighten and upset them. Or they may themselves become the targets. We all know children can be very irritating, sometimes deliberately, and often they do not know when to stop. But sometimes, the least little thing they do can provoke you. You shout at them, they cry, and you get more annoyed.

Because they are your children, your inhibitions may be lower, you lose your temper and strike out. Some women who normally would not dream of so much as slapping their children, lash out, often fiercely, under the influence of pre menstrual irritability.

This can be very upsetting for the mother as well as the children, as Rosemary found. You may remember that her husband left her because he found her pre menstrual moods impossible to handle.

'Recently I hit my three year old daughter. Although I felt extremely ashamed while it was happening, I also felt at the end of my tether and even a three hour walk in bad weather barely dampened the rage. But of course it subsided when bleeding started and I was left appalled at my behaviour – exhausted and hopeless.'

Helen, who has two children, found a similar problem.

'It starts about a week before my period. I get impossible with my children and hit them, not just slapping but really punching them. I am afraid that one day I am going to go too far. I tell myself at the time not to, but it is just as if I'm outside myself watching someone else do it.'

Sometimes, as we saw earlier, PMT only starts after the birth of your first child. This can be particularly unsettling because you have **two** new events to cope with at the same time. However much you wanted the baby, its arrival has an enormous impact on your life. You have to adjust to having a third member of the family, who is totally dependent on you, very time and energy consuming and always there.

At the same time, you find yourself becoming moody. You are depressed, or irritable, and you find that you get tired very easily. This only lasts for a few days each month, but, if you have never suffered from PMT before, you wonder what has got into you suddenly.

The baby becomes a burden instead of a pleasure. If the baby cries you become irritated, and when he will not stop you slap or shake him in a desperate attempt to quieten him down. Occasionally you may go too far. Like Sandra:

'I have suffered from mild PMT since I was eleven. But since I had the baby, I go berserk two weeks in four. Sometimes, it is all I can do not to kill her. I don't know what gets into me. I just keep hitting her, and it is very hard to stop.'

Like Sandra, many women feel that what they are doing is somehow out of their control. They have the frightening feeling that they are 'possessed'. Sometimes the injuries they inflict on their children are severe – several women have had to take their children to the doctor with severe bruising or broken limbs. Usually they find it impossible to admit to the doctor that they have inflicted these injuries and make up a plausible story instead. Obviously it is a very embarrassing and shameful thing to acknowledge, especially if you believe that it is bred of some deep seated malice or evil in you, as many women do. But there is a vicious circle. As long as you do not tell your doctor, he may not realise that there is anything wrong and so your problem goes untreated. But, unfortunately of course, some women who do tell their doctors get very unsympathetic treatment which only reinforces their shame and misery. PMT is not spotted, and so it is not treated.

As with so many areas of PMT, no research has been done into baby battering and its relationship to PMT. I am certainly not suggesting that **all** baby battering is caused by PMT. But there is a strong possibility that PMT is a contributory factor or the direct cause of much baby battering and is therefore something that should always be considered. Many women and their families have been helped by correct treatment for PMT (see Chapter Eleven), which has helped prevent a great deal of misery.

CASE HISTORY: MAUREEN

Maureen is now 46, married with one daughter, Lesley, aged 20. Maureen's PMT only started after the birth of Lesley.

'I started blowing up, my fingers and ankles, and it became hard to walk. And these awful headaches would start and drum in my head. I went to the doctor lots of times because of these bad heads. And I did tell him that my daughter was getting on my nerves and he just used to say: "Well, everybody has a child. You're not the only one. Pull yourself together." And this began to be a regular occurrence. It was always "Pull yourself together" and "You've only got one, other people have got two or three children".

'Well, I know it sounds callous, but I didn't really enjoy having a child. It didn't come easy. It seemed that everything I did was hard labour. I wasn't a very sympathetic mother.

'It nearly always seemed to be about mealtimes when Lesley would start getting me worked up. And then it would go from bad to worse. I would shout at her and she would cry and then I would shake her and hit her, even though she

6

was still only very tiny. I feel terribly guilty even now, remembering what I did. Once, when she was about five, I went into the bedroom and found her cutting the eiderdown up and blowing the feathers in the air. And we had saved a long time to get that eiderdown. Well, something seemed to snap. I gave her a swipe and picked her up and threw her across the room. I thought I had knocked her out. Fortunately, someone rang the door bell, otherwise I don't know what I would have done.

'The final straw came at Christmas time. I was really feeling wretched. In fact, I was feeling like murder, much more than Christmas. I hadn't even bought Lesley any toys and I wanted to be nasty. I wanted to tell her there wasn't a Father Christmas, nastiness was really taking over. And I didn't get any Christmas food in, or anything. Then I thought, I'll make one last effort and go to the doctor. Christmas time his surgery must be empty, he must listen to me. But it was the same thing. Nerve pills. Tranquillisers.

'All the way home I cried. In fact, I wanted to die. Then I saw a neighbour and she said: "Whatever is the matter with you? What are you crying for?" And I told her I'd been to the doctor again and got slimming pills, sleeping pills and what have you, everything again, and that I kept on feeling so awful around the time of my period. Well, she recommended me to a doctor who treated PMT, and I became a new woman.'

Lesley can remember much of her mother's anger and depression and, although they now get on very well together, she remembers her own fear at what was coming next.

'I didn't want to bring friends home in case Mum was in one of her moods. I used to lock myself in my room and insist that I was never coming out again. But really that only made things worse because as soon as I did come out Mum would storm into my room, hit me and grab my things and start ripping them up. The worst thing I remember is that she broke my guitar: I never did learn to play.

'As soon as Mum had received treatment, she started trying to make up to me and it was like having a new mother. She would meet me from school, buy me sweets and toys. As she says, she was trying to put herself in a good light in my eyes.'

Fortunately for Maureen and Lesley, treatment came in time to give them both a chance to get to know each other better in happier circumstances, and Lesley seems undamaged by her early experiences. When she was fifteen, she started to suffer herself from PMT.

'Mum was a terrific help. She spotted the signs in me; I did not realise it myself. But I remember feeling the whole world was against me sometimes, and I would sulk in my room, and not do my homework. My school reports got worse and worse, though I used to be quite good at school. I was due to take "O" levels when Mum finally insisted that I go to her doctor for treatment. It was amazing. I suddenly found that I did not go through ups and downs nearly so much, I found it much easier to concentrate on my work. I did quite well in my exams, in fact, and I'm sure that is thanks to the treatment.'

Maureen was able to put her own experience of PMT to good use and be understanding and supportive to Lesley when she needed it most.

Chapter Seven

Taking Yourself to Task

'Oh, ignore her if she is being difficult, it is just the time of the month.'

How often have you heard that said about yourself or another woman, usually by a man? It is a patronising and unsympathetic generalisation, based on ignorance and half truths, and makes the mistake of assuming that, because **some** women have been seen to behave strangely around the time of their period, **all** women do.

But now that women are going out to work in increasingly large numbers, the question is becoming more pertinent: does the cyclical flow of your hormones affect your ability to perform and cope with a regular job? When PMT is raised as a subject, it is often assumed that the mere existence of the menstrual cycle means that women will automatically be erratic and so cannot be relied on to hold down a regular job. Worse, the assumption is that, because PMT exists, all women must be prone to it.

Several studies have now been done to see whether women in general, as opposed to those known to suffer from PMT are affected by the menstrual cycle. Tests have been carried out to check their speed of response in certain situations, their reflexes, their powers of concentration, their ability to perform repetitive tasks accurately. Different surveys have come to different conclusions. Some found that there is absolutely no difference in performance by women at any particular stage of their menstrual cycle. Others concluded that the menstrual cycle does make some difference to some women's ability to perform certain tasks. The problem with these tests was that they looked at all women. They did not isolate women who suffered from PMT and test only them.

But at least there is one clear and reassuring conclusion to be drawn: there are no grounds for assuming that, because all women have menstrual cycles, all women will vary considerably in their abilities during the course of a month.

With many women their fluctuating hormones appear to have little if any effect on their moods, or their health, and consequently have no bearing on their ability to tackle a job. Other women who do suffer from PMT experience only very mild symptoms, like a slight tendency to swelling or tender breasts. A symptom which incapacitates you in one job may affect you less seriously in another. Bloatedness, for instance, might be enough to significantly affect your performance in sport. On its own, however, it would probably have very little effect on your ability as an administrator or teacher.

But the fact remains that, for those who do suffer from severe PMT, there can be problems which we should recognise. For if we deny them, we are encouraging the ignorance and neglect of PMT that has existed for far too long already. The answer is to treat the problem and then it won't be a problem any more.

Work

All the symptoms of PMT can affect the way you feel about your job and your ability to cope with it. It may take an extra effort on your part, in the week prior to your period, not to let the strains show. Errors may creep into routine tasks and you may be much less tolerant of your own or other people's mistakes. Louise, an executive in a consumer organisation, was usually very calm and efficient, but she suffered from severe pre menstrual headaches which made her work a burden sometimes:

'Often it was all I could do not to scream "leave me

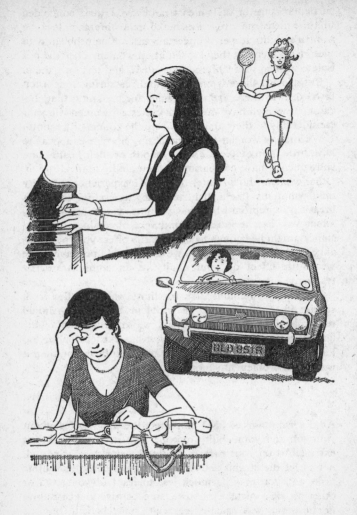

alone" and throw all my papers in the air as I ran crying from the room. But somehow, I'd manage to hang on. I'd try to avoid meetings and postpone important decision making during my pre menstrual week, but of course that was not always possible.'

Talking to many working women who suffer from PMT, it is clear that most of them, like Louise, make a special effort to keep going no matter how bad they feel, and do their best to hide the fact of their suffering from their colleagues. Often this means bottling up feelings at work which then erupt more violently and painfully once they get home.

Sandra works as a reporter for a local radio station in Illinois. 'I get very irritable before my periods, but obviously I can't afford to let this show too much at work, particularly when I'm interviewing someone on air. So I bite back my irritation as much as I can during the day and shamelessly take it out on my long-suffering partner when I get home. I hate myself for being like this but each month, no matter how hard I try, the same thing happens. Sometimes it makes my work a tremendous strain and I have to admit that it does suffer then. But I think I make up for that by the extra energy I put into it during the rest of the month.'

Different jobs bring different problems. One popular actress found her lines much harder to learn during her pre menstrual week, and never felt that she gave her best performances during that time 'unless the part required me to weep, which I could manage very easily!' She used to dread auditions prior to her period. Feeling tense and uncomfortable anyway, her fear of failing was intensified.

Costumes were a problem too. If she had a fitting during her good weeks but had to wear the costume in the week before her period it would be uncomfortably tight and sometimes didn't fit at all. Once she had treatment for PMT she found that she was more relaxed throughout the month and her costumes were comfortable too!

Paula Weideger, in her book 'Menstruation and Menopause' tells the story of a friend of hers who was having singing lessons regularly. One day her teacher asked her if she was coming up to her period by any chance. She was in fact due to start the following day. 'I thought so,' he said. 'The quality of your voice is not as good as usual.' It is quite common for this to happen. There is sometimes a loss of muscle control during the pre menstrual period and this can affect the quality of voice control. Someone with a trained ear can clearly hear the difference.

Anything that is particularly testing can be an extra strain if it falls on a day when you are suffering from PMT. Job interviews are a good example of this. As one woman wrote:

'I have to find a job and am extremely worried about the timing of the hoped-for interviews, because in the week before my period my ability to present myself diminishes sharply. Apart from a general appearance of unassertiveness, I can go totally blank or burst into tears. I know I always manage one way or another, but it is dreadful feeling so impotent.'

Examinations are another example. They are bad enough at any time, but they can be worse if you are suffering from PMT. Dr Dalton has shown that school-girls do less well in exams that they take during their pre menstrual time. Several women remember that they dreaded exams falling in their pre menstrual week because they found it harder to concentrate and felt generally more 'under the weather' at that time.

Often, no one realises the connection. It is very rare for students to be given the chance to mention that they are suffering from PMT on the day of an important exam. Yet the result could have a crucial affect on their career. Obviously, this is open to abuse – PMT, especially for children, could be the all embracing excuse that covers a multitude of sins. But that should not be used to ride rough-shod over legitimate problems they may have.

It is like refusing to admit that poor eyesight can affect your ability to see a blackboard, or your driving or your tennis playing. You do not have to stop doing any of these things – you get glasses to help you do them as well as any-one else.

In the same way, if you suffer from severe PMT, you do not have to stop working, you just need treatment.

Many women find that they feel at their most resourceful and dynamic in midcycle and notice that they seem to accomplish more and with more success at that time of the month. Sometimes, this burst of energy comes just before the onset of PMT.

Lydia, a scriptwriter for a large television studio is like that, 'It's amazing, about a week before my period I get an incredible surge of energy – it's almost obsessive. I know that it is the best time to get things done and clear my desk.'

Accidents

PMT, it seems, can play an important part in causing accidents. In a survey of accidents among women in five

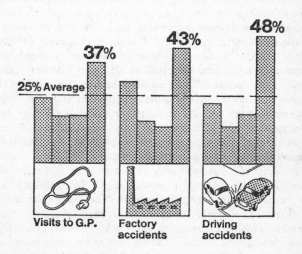

Timing of accidents in relation to the menstrual cycle.
(Month is divided into four weeks starting with the onset of menstruation.)

light engineering factories, it was found that 43% of the accidents occurred to women in their pre menstrual week. Similar indications of increased clumsiness and lack of concentration emerged from a survey of London hospitals by Dr Dalton. She found that half of all emergency admissions occurred during the pre menstrual week. Interestingly, this applied to all areas of the hospital, from medical emergencies like strokes, through surgical emergencies like appendicitis, to infections, fevers or admissions to psychiatric wards.

A report by the Medical Committee on Accident Prevention confirmed these findings. They studied accident admissions to hospitals in the Wolverhampton area, and attendances at doctors' surgeries. In both cases, they found a significantly higher number of accidents occurred to women in their pre menstrual week.

The US Centre for Safety Education has shown that the 48 hours before the onset of a period is a woman's most dangerous and most vulnerable time, when accidents at work are more likely to occur. The same, of course, is likely to be true for accidents at home, though no studies have been done to confirm this. Indeed, although I do not know how many, some of the hospital accident admissions I mentioned earlier may well have happened at home. One woman told me that she sprained her ankle six times in the course of a year. On checking back on the dates of her visit to the doctor, she found that all her sprains had occurred in the week prior to her period!

It seems too, that you may have a reduced resistance to infection during your pre menstrual days. This explains why, as we saw at the start, you have an increased chance of ending up in hospital at that time. In fact, several doctors now recommend that women who are due for major surgery avoid going into hospital during the week prior to their periods because their recovery rate may be slower then, and there is an increased chance of contracting an additional, and potentially very dangerous, infection.

Car accidents are another hazard for sufferers of severe PMT. The Medical Committee on Accident Prevention found that nearly half, (48%) of the accidents had occurred when the women were in their pre menstrual week, much higher than the average 25% you would normally expect in any one week of four. Surprisingly, this applied not only to women drivers, but also to women passengers, perhaps because their reactions were slower and so they did not brace themselves well for the impact of the crash. Several women have mentioned that they notice that their driving is more erratic just before their period. Christine, a young doctor, had seven bumps and scrapes in her car in 18 months, always in the week prior to her period. Joan, a teacher, would not drive her car if she could avoid it during her pre menstrual week:

'My concentration went completely, and I'd forget to indicate when I was turning, silly but important things like that. I also became very irritable and tense, to the point that if I was caught in a traffic jam, it was all I could do not to deliberately run into a car in front in frustration. I think my reactions were slower, too, and I found myself braking sharply all the time, narrowly avoiding an accident. Frankly, I didn't feel safe driving with myself at that time!'

Now that Joan has had treatment for PMT, she is back on the road with confidence.

Lack of concentration, lethargy and slower reaction time are probably some of the main reasons why many accidents occur pre menstrually. It is also likely that you are clumsier and less co-ordinated, all of which can lead to injuries. Mood swings can contribute too, of course. If you are feeling irritable, you may become more aggressive and drive more recklessly or perform tasks at work without observing all the safety precautions. If you are depressed, your alertness may well be diminished.

Crime and Punishment

Statistics gathered among women prisoners show that more women commit crimes during their pre menstrual week than at any other time. A survey of 156 newly convicted women prisoners in Britain showed that almost half (49%) had committed their crime in the four days before their period or the first four days of their period. Of the women who knew they suffered from PMT, well over half (63%) of them had committed the crime during the time of their symptoms. In another study on women in prison, Morton found that 62% of crimes of violence by women had been committed in their pre menstrual week compared with only 2% in the first week after menstruation.

The reason for these findings is probably not that you are more likely to commit a crime during your pre menstrual week. The more probable explanation is that lack of concentration and tension makes you clumsier, less wary and slower to react and so more likely to be caught.

Treatment can make a tremendous difference. In Westfield State Prison in America, Dr Morton and colleagues experimented by treating women prisoners who suffered from PMT. They found that, as a result, the women behaved better, felt better, and so received fewer punishments and that there was a general rise in their morale.

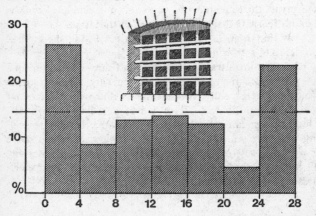

Timing of offences by women during the menstrual cycle.

(Month is divided into four day periods starting with the onset of menstruation. Dotted line indicates expected incidence on a statistical basis.)

In fact, I cannot stress too much that if you are a PMT sufferer you should treat the problem at its root. Obviously you will work and feel better once you have PMT under control.

Sport

Ann Hayden Jones, the former Wimbledon tennis champion, has suffered from PMT since she first started her periods. Her symptoms are sometimes quite severe, and hard to cope with for a top tennis player.

'When I started playing tennis seriously I would never admit that I suffered from PMT. That would be like telling your opponent your weakest stroke. But I certainly felt the effect. For one thing, playing became more of an effort and I'd find it harder to get myself into the right frame of mind before a match. I used to feel heavy and lethargic – chasing the ball was more of an effort – my reactions were slower and the tension I always felt during a match would be much more intense.

'I was shorter tempered too. When things went wrong, or if there were doubtful line calls, I would be furious when suffering from PMT whereas usually I took things like that in my stride. And being angry often affected my game, for the worse.

'Another odd thing I noticed was that I couldn't judge the ball as well as usual – PMT seemed to put my "eye" out. Other women tennis players have told me that they find the same thing.'

A young woman doctor I know, who plays a fine game of squash, began to find she was missing easy shots and losing games she expected to win. When she checked she found that her loss of form always occurred during her pre menstrual week. It is in fact quite common for athletes to alter their menstrual cycle with the contraceptive pill in order to avoid PMT and to defer menstruation, because some women find that their performance also suffers while they are actually bleeding.

Ann Hayden Jones says that she had to be very deter-

mined not to let PMT become an excuse for poor performance, because one lost match can put you out of a vital
tournament.

'I suppose there are some women who don't fight it and
let it get the better of them. But I wanted to succeed so I
made sure PMT didn't stop me. But it certainly was a
struggle at times. I think it is definitely harder for a woman
than for a man to cope with the pressures of the tennis
circuit.'

It is not hard to find the reasons why PMT would have an
adverse effect on the performance of sportswomen. All the
symptoms like water retention, lack of concentration,
clumsiness, lethargy would obviously take their toll. But
sports are also a special case because they are based on
competition and success at reaching certain targets. It is
soon clear whether you are doing well or not.

Sports also highlight the positive side of the menstrual
cycle, which is often forgotten. Research by the Women's
Amateur Athletic Association showed that the majority of
women athletes give their best performances during the two
weeks immediately following their periods, at midcycle in
fact. Other studies have indicated that women have an
increased spirit of competitiveness at this time. This is not
necessarily the same thing as feelings of aggression that
many women experience in their pre menstrual week. Then
the aggression is often negative, based on tension, irritability
and feelings of frustration at being less able to cope. Competitiveness is generally a positive feeling, based on a sense
of your own abilities and your own worth, the feeling that
you can triumph whatever the odds.

If you suffer from bad PMT you would probably decide
against a sporting career. Sportswomen are generally, as you
would expect, those women least afflicted by physical ailments of all sorts, not just PMT.

So, it is not altogether surprising that women have won
top sporting titles both while menstruating and during their
pre menstrual week. They clearly do not suffer from PMT
and in fact confirm what we said at the beginning of this
chapter, that it is totally unfair to blame all women's

problems on PMT. If, in sport, where performance is easily measured, many women do consistently well throughout their cycle, it is reasonable to assume that in other areas other women who do not suffer from PMT are equally consistent.

Chapter Eight

The Final Straw

I was talking to a friend of mine and I mentioned that I was writing a book about PMT. It turned out, as it so often has, that she is a sufferer.

'PMT wouldn't be so bad if it wasn't for one thing – the depression. As if life wasn't hard enough anyway! Already I'm moving house and changing jobs. Now, to top it all I'm feeling bloated, tense and so miserable. It just doesn't seem fair.' And my usually placid friend burst into tears.

Many women find that depression is the worst part of PMT. The physical symptoms can be depressing enough in themselves, even if you do not suffer too badly. But to these is often added a general feeling of misery, which is one of the most common symptoms of PMT.

Of course, there is depression and depression. At its mildest you may become more tearful and unsettled, likely to swing from cheerfulness to tears within the space of five minutes. That can be disconcerting and inconvenient but it is not the end of the world, and usually passes quite quickly.

On the other hand, like my friend, you may be a sunny, calm person going through a stressful time, and PMT makes this a lot worse. You might be having difficulties at work, or one of your children is getting into trouble at school, or a much loved elderly relative has a long-term illness you have to tend. PMT will make anything like this much harder to cope with. It does not happen in isolation, just once, like measles, when you can put yourself to bed, take a dose of medicine and lap up the tea and sympathy. It comes on top of everything else, regularly as clockwork, once a month. Then, with worries as well, the onset of PMT and depression can be the last straw. Or you may be nervous and highly-strung, with a high level of anxiety. Small things worry you and you feel tense, stressed and miserable on and off throughout the month. With the onset of PMT as well, you may become severely depressed.

Obviously PMT has not caused these feelings, but it does make them worse at the critical time each month. Then anxieties become deep worries, misery turns to depression and you cannot see how your life can ever sort itself out again.

Of course, depression can be an illness in its own right that affects you at any time, not just before your period. And men suffer from depression, too, although in general nearly twice as many women as men are sufferers. Depression can be caused by many things from the more obvious, like the loss of someone you love, to complicated psychological stresses which may even date from your childhood.

Depression is often described as a sense of loss, but that can mean a lot of things. One of the best descriptions is 'the self seems worthless, the outer world meaningless and the future hopeless'. In other words, you lose faith in yourself, nothing you do seems to go right and you can see no light at the end of the tunnel.

A sad event, like the death of someone you love, or the breaking up of an important relationship, can trigger off these feelings, though it is important to separate depression from grief. We all feel grief and pain when something like that happens in our lives, that is a natural and necessary reaction. But we do get over it. There may be a lingering sense of loss, and there may be moments when we weep quietly again over what has happened, but we do not dwell on it, and eventually the unhappiness passes. If it persists, if you cannot shake off the grief, then the natural sorrow may become depression and the depression becomes serious.

As we have already seen with PMT generally, depression

can spread into other aspects of your life. It can make you apathetic and lazy or you may feel unloving and unloved. Things, and sometimes even people, who were important to you suddenly lose their value. Your marriage, your relationships, your work can all suffer.

How do you distinguish between general depression, mild or severe, and the depression caused by PMT. The only clear test is **when** you feel depressed. If you feel so miserable only in the week or ten days before your period, then clearly the depression is linked with PMT. Rita, who is a dental assistant, realised the connection between her periods and her depression because of a chance remark by one of her colleagues. He had noticed that she had been very depressed on his birthday: she had tried to be cheerful, but it was obviously an effort. The following month, she was just the same and he noticed that it was almost exactly one month after his birthday. He mentioned this to Rita, she checked up and found she always seemed to feel depressed just before her periods. Finding this out was a great relief to her, because she had begun to think that she was a 'natural depressive'.

Another point to watch for is whether general feelings of depression get worse at the same time each month, in the days before your period. If it is then that the intolerable black moods descend, your depression is not caused by, but is clearly increased by the overload of PMT. Taking away the PMT may not solve all your problems but it will certainly make life easier.

If you are depressed, it is tempting to believe that PMT is at the root of all your depression. Treat that, you may think, and all my misery will go away. Well, you may be lucky. In Rita's case, treating her PMT did relieve her depression. Of course she still felt miserable sometimes, as we all do, but she did not get the sense that she could never be happy again.

But treating PMT will not suddenly sort out all the other areas of your life too. If circumstances are difficult, or you are suffering from depression unrelated to your period, none of these will miraculously go away along with your PMT.

But, and it is a very important but, relieving your PMT will lift one burden from you and this can make the others considerably easier to bear.

Finding a Way Out

We all have our own ways of trying to lift the gloom of depression. Friends or family can be a great help by lending a sympathetic and understanding ear. But sometimes it is difficult to talk about it, even to them. Instead, some women try taking pills, like aspirin or tranquillisers, to ease the misery. These may dull your senses temporarily but, as tranquillisers are depressants themselves, they can sometimes make things worse. If your depression is related to PMT they do little to relieve your symptoms.

Jackie, who is twenty-five with two small children, had been taking tranquillisers for some time because her doctor did not realise that her depression was connected with PMT and was at his wits end to know what to do.

'It wasn't his fault. I mean, I didn't realise that the depressions hit me regularly each month. But the pills didn't help at all. They just turned me into a zombie, or more of a zombie to be exact, because I used to get a bit sloppy and vague as well before I started taking the pills. But the tranquillisers seemed to make me feel twenty times worse. I can't tell you the difference it made when it was discovered I was suffering from PMT and I got treatment for that. I still get depressed, I think it's the way I am, but not every month and I come out of it again and it doesn't get worse each month now like it used to.'

* * *

Some women turn to alcohol to relieve symptoms of anxiety, tension, frustration and depression – in other words, to cheer themselves up. 'Drowning your sorrows in drink' is a well known expression, but it can have a nasty twist for PMT sufferers. If you are aware of when your periods are due you may have already noticed, even if you are not a heavy drinker, that one glass is enough to set your head reeling during your pre menstrual week. This is because, just as your tissues are more ready to retain water, so they are equally ready to retain alcohol, and it is absorbed much more quickly and fully, with increased effect.

You may be aware of this, and cut down your drinking accordingly. But if you are drinking because you feel depressed and need consolation, then you may not want, or be able, to stop. You may notice that the drink is having a greater effect than usual and, before you know where you are, you are getting 'woozy' or even drunk.

A vicious circle may start. You feel more depressed and despairing before your period, so you drink for temporary relief. You may drink too much, become drunk quite easily and then find it hard to know when to stop. Since alcohol in the long term is a depressant, anxiety-producing, addictive drug, you may find over-drinking becoming a regular monthly routine and the gradual slide into alcoholism begins.

In a survey done in America, 67% of women alcoholics related their drinking bouts to their menstrual cycle and all of them felt that their drinking had begun or increased during the pre menstrual period. Clinics that specialise in the treatment of alcoholism frequently notice that women alcoholics who come to them for help drink more heavily in the week before their periods. They have also found that women are more likely to go back to drinking, after a period of remaining 'dry', during their pre menstrual week. The extra strains of PMT sap their willpower, make them more miserable and they turn to drink to cheer themselves up.

ACCEPT, Britain's largest alcoholism clinic, based in London, treats many women problem drinkers. They hold regular group sessions to make women more aware of the pressures of PMT. They point out your 'vulnerability periods', in particular the 10 days or so before your period.

As Charles Vetter, the clinic director, put it: 'If you know when the pressures that cause you to drink are likely to occur, you have a much better chance of preparing yourself. So we get women to keep a diary of their drinking bouts and their periods, and we find time and again that they tie up. A whole cluster of problems which a woman might have coped with till then, suddenly become too much for her and she starts drinking in desperation, hoping to relieve her miseries. We had one woman, for example, who had 7 relapses. She kept a diary and it turned out that they each occurred in the 3 or 4 days before her period.'

In view of all this it is hardly surprising that in a British jail it was found that a high proportion of women taken into custody for assault or drunk and disorderly behaviour were about to start their periods.

* * *

Sometimes the pre menstrual period can be more dangerous than you expect or bargain for. At its worst, depression can lead you to such despair that you feel the only way out is to end it all. Sheila suffered from severe pre menstrual depression for ten years.

'Sometimes I got so depressed I just wanted to die. Once it got so bad that I grabbed hold of a bottle of tablets my husband was taking and swallowed the lot. Luckily they found me before it was too late.'

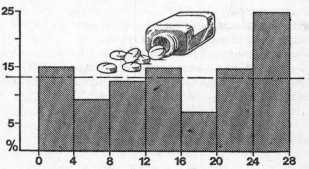

Number of suicide attempts in relation to menstrual cycle.
(Month is divided into four day periods starting with the onset of menstruation. Dotted line indicates expected incidence on a statistical basis.)

Sheila actually made an attempt to commit suicide. Many women get no further than thinking about it. Others not only attempt suicide, they succeed. Several studies in Britain and America have shown that many more women attempt to commit suicide, or do commit suicide, in the days before their period than at any other time of the month. That is a frightening fact which makes the recognition and understanding of PMT all the more urgent.

I am not suggesting that PMT **causes** suicides but it clearly contributes to them. As I said at the beginning of this chapter, depression can stem from many things, and PMT is just one of these. How depressed you feel in your pre menstrual days will very much depend on the circumstances of your life and your personality – in other words, how depressed you feel at other times of the month – as well as how severely you get PMT. It is one thing to say you want to commit suicide and quite another to do it. The women who go to that extreme are almost certainly women who are depressed for other reasons, but PMT adds the extra load of misery that they cannot stand. The combination of the physical problems of PMT, the psychological mood changes and, above all, the depression may tip the balance. The feeling, very common with depression, that it will never go away again, may become so strong under the pressure of PMT that ending it all seems the only way out.

Realising that you suffer from PMT, and doing something about it, will not necessarily stop you feeling suicidal. But it might make enough difference to hold you back from such a drastic step. That is the important thing.

CASE HISTORY: CLAIRE

Claire is 32, single and a secretary. She started suffering from PMT when she was about 14 years old.

'I went to the doctor and he said, "It's just one of those things, dear, you'll be all right when you have had babies" and he wouldn't give me anything.

'As I got older, my PMT seemed to get worse. I was

really an extraordinary person before my period. I don't know how my boyfriends put up with me – in fact, I always seemed to split up with them just before my period. I wasn't very good with girlfriends, either, and wouldn't go out or see them for about ten days before my period. Then I would become quite a nice, friendly person again for the rest of the month.

'At 19 I started drinking heavily and definitely more when my period was coming up, though I didn't realise the connection at the time. I just felt I needed a pick-me-up because I used to be so down and edgy. This developed into a big drinking problem and I was definitely drinking alcoholically.

'I have been to hospital four times to dry out and each time they asked me as a routine question, when my period was due. And each time it has been due right then, and started either the day I went to hospital or the day after. My relapses were just the same – always in the days before my period.

'I know that for sure because I have always kept a regular diary. Looking back over it, it was obvious that I drank more during the days I suffered PMT. I've written things like "edgy all day" or "had a row with John" and "slept badly, woke up feeling grim" and "panicked and bought a bottle of Vodka" on consecutive days and then the next day "started my period" – and it is like that all through my diary.

'Twice I have felt so awful before my period, depressed and desperate, that I have tried to kill myself. Once I took some tablets but they found me in time. About a year later, I tried to cut my wrist with a razor blade but I couldn't bear to watch what I was doing and so I stopped before I'd done any very serious damage. Both times, my period started the day after.

'It was the alcoholic clinic I went to that suggested the connection between my periods and my drinking bouts, and of course my diaries showed they were right. But I don't blame PMT for my drinking, or my suicide attempts. I just think that PMT was the last straw. It seemed to come on top of all my other problems and magnify them so I felt there was no escape.'

Two years ago Claire received treatment for her PMT and she has not touched alcohol since then.

'I've gained confidence since I started treatment and stopped drinking. I go out much more now and I've joined a ballet class, something I would never have dared to do before. I'm much less aggressive now, more gentle, and so much happier. It is really like a miracle: I feel well all the time for the first time in my life.'

Chapter Nine

Have You Really Got PMT?

As I have said before, there is only one way to find out if you really are suffering from PMT. You need to chart when your symptoms occur to see if there is a regular pattern each month – symptoms in the week or ten days before your period, free of symptoms the rest of the time.

To make sure your symptoms **are** connected with your periods, it is worth keeping a menstrual chart for two or three months. The pattern will soon show up if you are suffering from PMT. This will help you to see when to expect your symptoms and, if you go to a doctor, it could be a very important first step in convincing him to take you seriously.

Over the page you will see what a menstrual chart looks like when it has been filled in. You mark your symptoms in the square opposite the day they occurred. Most women have symbols they use for different things like H for headaches, M for migraine, B for bloatedness and so on. If several symptoms start on the same day and you have not got room to fill them all in one square, you could just mark down S for symptoms and make a note of what they are in the margin or on a separate piece of paper.

Mark in too the days that you have your periods, perhaps with P. If you are suffering from PMT you should be able to see a regular pattern arising each month, with a cluster of symptoms occurring in the days before your period and completely symptom-free days immediately after your

	May	June	July	Aug.
1				
2				
3				
4				
5				
6				
7				H
8		H		H
9		T		H+T
10		M		H+T
11		M	H+B	P
12		T	H+B	P
13		T	H+B	P
14	H+B	P	H+T	P
15	H+B	P	P	
16	H+T	P	P	
17	H+T	P	P	
18	H			
19	P			
20	P			
21	P			
22	P			
23				
24				
25				
26				
27				
28				
29				
30				
31				

B = bloatedness
M = migraine
T = tension
H = headache
P = period

A menstrual chart which has been filled in by a PMT sufferer

1				
2				
3				
4				
5				
6				
7				
8				
9				
10				
11				
12				
13				
14				
15				
16				
17				
18				
19				
20				
21				
22				
23				
24				
25				
26				
27				
28				
29				
30				
31				

A menstrual chart for you to fill in

period. You will see what I mean if you look at the completed chart. You will also find a blank menstrual chart for you to fill in yourself.

If you keep a diary, it is also worth looking back through it and making charts for previous months, marking in symptoms where you can remember them. The more months you can show, the more convincing the pattern of your symptoms will be.

Symptom Score Chart

St Thomas's Hospital have prepared a different chart, designed to show the severity of your symptoms. If you are planning to go to a doctor it might be a good idea to fill that in too so that you have a clear record of which symptoms affect you most. You simply mark on the symptom score chart, the day of the cycle when your symptoms started and ended and put a tick to indicate how severe they each were. One tick = mild, two ticks = unpleasant but not extreme, three ticks = very unpleasant. The first day of your period is Day One, so you would expect your symptoms to start from about Day Twenty onwards, as a rough guide.

Record your symptoms for at least one and preferably two menstrual cycles. You can do this in conjunction with a menstrual chart so that you show not only the timing of your symptoms but their severity. Day One is the first day of your period.

Symptom	Day of Cycle Start	End	Severity of symptoms: 3 – very troublesome 2 – unpleasant but not extreme 1 – mild
Depression			
Irritability			/
Anxiety, tension			
Lethargy			
Lack of co-ordination (clumsiness, accidents)			
Breast tenderness			
Swollen abdomen			
Swollen ankles or fingers			
Headaches			
Migraine			
Food cravings			
Aches and pains, backache			
Lack of concentration			
Other symptoms			

Finally, here is a check-list of symptoms. These are the main symptoms from which you are likely to suffer, divided into groups for convenience. You will probably find that you suffer from several of the symptoms in different groups. This should provide a handy reference for you. If you are suffering from something that does **not** appear in this list it is unlikely that it is a symptom of PMT.

Check-List of Symptoms

Physical changes

Weight gain	Dizziness, faintness	Backache
Skin disorders	Cold sweats	General aches
Painful breasts	Nausea, sickness	and pains
Swelling	Hot flushes	
Eye diseases	Fuzzy vision	
Asthma	Spontaneous bruising	
Epilepsy	Headache, migraine	

Concentration

Sleeplessness	Lowered judgement	Lack of
Forgetfulness	Difficulty	Coordination
Confusion	concentrating	
	Accidents	

Behaviour changes

Lowered school	Stay at home	Food cravings
or work	Avoid social	Drinking too
performance	activities	much alcohol
Lethargy	Decreased efficiency	Taking too
		many pills

Mood changes

Mood swings	Restlessness	Tension
Crying	Irritability	Loss of
Depression	Aggression	sex drive
Anxiety		

Chapter Ten

Helping Yourself

There are three golden rules for coping with PMT:

1. REDUCE STRESS ON YOURSELF.

2. BUILD UP YOUR DEFENCES.

3. ALLEVIATE YOUR SYMPTOMS AND TREAT THE CAUSE.

In this chapter I will try to help you put these rules into practice. But, before I do, a word of caution. If you suffer only mildly, then a few sensible changes in diet and routine may be all you need to help yourself. Even if your symptoms are more severe, there are many ways you can make PMT easier to bear. But don't expect to achieve miracles on your own. As we saw earlier, there are basic physical causes of PMT which may need specific treatment that only your doctor can prescribe. If you find that, after all you do, your PMT is still unbearable, you need and should seek your doctor's help.

But, **this chapter will make life easier for you.** If your doctor is unsympathetic, it may help to tide you over until you can find a doctor who will treat you. If you are starting treatment, it may help you until the cure works. If you are the type of woman who avoids doctors and tablets whenever possible, you want perhaps to try to help yourself first. And if your symptoms are mild it may be all the help you need.

Get to know yourself

Before you do anything else, check that you really are suffering from PMT. To do that, look at the symptom chart (see page 110) and see how your symptoms compare. We have divided them into categories, so that you can see **how** you suffer. Do you find that most of your symptoms fall into the physical categories? Or do you suffer more from the psychological symptoms?

Understanding the way in which PMT affects you can make it easier for you to sort out ways of helping yourself. And if you go to the doctor, it can help him to choose the most suitable treatment for you.

You should also keep a menstrual chart for two or three months, as we suggested in Chapter Nine. That way you will know when PMT affects you. And seeing the pattern of your PMT will help you to take action against it.

Tell the family

Forewarned is forearmed. Once you know when and how PMT will affect you, all those aches and pains, and outbursts of tears or temper are fairly predictable. As it is most often the family, the people you live with, who have to bear the brunt of your moods, you should make sure that they know the reason for and the timing of your symptoms.

One woman used to keep a calendar in the kitchen on which she marked BE CAREFUL in big letters in the week she expected PMT to strike. That way, both she and her family were prepared. As she told me:

'Often we'd forget all about it. Then a row started, usually with my husband or eldest son. Almost every time, one or other of us would catch sight of the calendar and there it was – BE CAREFUL. We ended up laughing together at how predictable I was.'

If your family are aware of PMT and what it can involve, they can help and support you. Talk about it with them, show them this book, share the experience. They may never have heard of it or thought about it before. Of course, just because they understand your problems, will not stop them shouting back when you argue, nor stop them irritating or upsetting you at times. But at least they won't be baffled by your changed personality and they may make efforts to keep their tempers in check, or to keep out of your way.

Sonia, who is fourteen, soon worked out a system of coping once her mother explained what was wrong:

'I always avoided mummy when she was in one of her pre menstrual moods. Everything I did seemed wrong so I was better off keeping out of her way. Somehow, even though we still had rows, it did help to know that it happened for a reason and that she was better and more fun the rest of the time.'

David, Sonia's father, avoided discussing important matters with his wife during her pre menstrual days.

'Most things can wait a few days, and I knew I'd get a much more considered view from her when she was not feeling tense and edgy.'

Other families know that it is best not to ask any favours at this time, or to expect extra help. On the contrary, some go out of their way to be extra kind and considerate instead. For instance, John and his son Tim have always helped around the house but make a special effort when Sheila has PMT. Taking your family into your confidence should help to avoid some of the worst clashes and will probably bring relief to you all.

Get organised

Organise, or rather re-organise your life to make things as easy as possible when PMT is due. After all, it is worth remembering that most of the month is trouble free.

Obviously, housework, your job, looking after the children and your family all have to go on, but you should be able to plan your time so that most difficulties – the predictable ones anyway – are sorted out and dealt with before those crucial few days.

For example, if you are at home looking after the house,

try to get the bulk of the housework done when you are feeling fine. Accept the fact that the house may not be quite so spotless during your pre menstrual days: that is not the end of the world! Plan meals and cook ahead as much as you can, too. And involve your husband and children in the shopping and running the house. Many husbands volunteer to do the cooking during that time once they know what is wrong.

Others look after the children in the evening, or help with baby's feed or nappy change. Peter, whose wife Brenda suffers from severe PMT, finds that his extra involvement with the baby is a huge bonus. 'It's silly but I'm not sure I would have done so much for the baby if it wasn't for Brenda's PMT – and yet I love every minute with the baby.'

If you are likely to put on weight pre menstrually, make sure you have clothes that fit you then. You will not look good squeezed into a dress that is obviously too tight and you certainly will not feel good. If your breasts swell, do not be afraid to get a larger bra, or one with a larger cup size. Try to avoid wearing tight girdles or clothes that constrict you. PMT is uncomfortable enough without making it worse!

At work, try to avoid fixing important meetings or visits when you know your period is coming up. If you are offered a choice, pick the time when you know you will feel better. You may be surprised at how easily people will adapt to your schedule, and how many routine tasks can be re-arranged to suit you.

In general, try not to get yourself into situations which will tax you. Don't invite friends round for dinner and don't accept invitations out if you don't feel up to it. But sometimes close friends can be a help, cheering you up and taking you out of yourself for a while. If you suffer aches and pains, don't make your pre menstrual week the one you decide to clear out all the cupboards. If you suffer emotional ups and downs, don't agree to have sixteen children over for a tea party. You know better than anyone what provokes you and what your symptoms are. A little bit of sensible thought and planning in your good weeks can make your bad days much easier to bear, for you and everyone you come into contact with.

Eat well

Making sure you eat well is about the best advice I can give you. It seems obvious enough, but it is amazing how many women skip meals or pick at their food at exactly the moment when they need nourishment most.

In fact, it is not hard to understand why. If you are feeling sick, tense and miserable, the chances are that the very thought of food makes you feel ill. But if you give into those feelings and do not eat, or if you go without food all day and just have one big meal at night, you will only make yourself feel worse. As we have already seen, lack of food can increase headaches and may even bring on a migraine attack.

The secret is to eat little and often. That way, your body is nourished throughout the day and you do not have to face large quantities of food all at once. Even if you do not feel like anything, try to make yourself eat at least some toast and a cup of tea or coffee, or a couple of biscuits. You will probably be surprised at how much better you feel afterwards. If you find that you often wake up in the morning feeling awful, a light snack just before you go to bed at night might help by keeping your body nourished while you are asleep.

Certain foods can be particularly good for you while you are suffering from PMT. You will remember that pyridoxine (Vitamin B6) plays an important role in the menstrual cycle. Some foods are particularly rich in Vitamin B6 along with other B vitamins: meat, particularly liver, milk, eggs as well as cereals, wholemeal bread, rice and yeast.

If you feel lethargic with PMT, then a high protein diet should give you more energy. Try to include a generous supply of meat, fish, milk, eggs or nuts in meals, or as a snack each day. You may also need a potassium boost, especially if you are taking diuretics. Bananas, tomatoes and orange juice are good sources of potassium, or you can buy potassium tablets at your local chemist shop. But too much potassium can have harmful side effects, so don't overdo it.

Coffee, black or white, dandelion leaves, parsley, watercress, celery juice and cucumber, are all mild natural diuretics which might help you to get rid of some of the extra water your tissues retain. It is also worth cutting down on the amount of liquid you drink so that you only have four or five cups a day during your pre menstrual days. Limit your salt intake too, because as you probably know, salt encourages your body to hold water.

If you suffer from stomach cramps some people, notably Adele Davis, believe that calcium can be very soothing. Milk eggs and cheese are all calcium-rich foods. The main thing is to make sure you eat a well balanced diet, with a good mixture of vitamins, carbohydrates, proteins and fats. There are several good books to help you choose the foods to eat and we recommend some at the end of this chapter.

If you are dieting, don't worry!

With your tissues soaked with water, you feel heavy and bloated, the scales resolutely refuse to go down and you feel sure your diet is not working. In a drastic attempt to keep to your weight loss, you start skipping meals only to find that you feel worse and you do not get any thinner.

It is very unfair on women that, while men can diet steadily all the time, many women have about one week in four when they cannot seem to lose weight no matter what they do. Even women who do not suffer much with PMT often find that their weight obstinately refuses to diminish because their water-weight is sufficient to counter any dieting they do.

The important thing is to realise what is happening so that it does not catch you out. Otherwise, if you do miss the connection with your period, you may become demoralised and depressed and begin to stuff yourself for comfort. Then, of course, you will gain fat, not just water, and that will be much harder to lose once your period starts. A vicious circle

116

sets up. Fierce dieting for three weeks, stuffing for one week, fierce dieting again and so on until your poor body does not know whether it is coming or going.

To avoid that, be aware of your body's cycles. When the scales stick, don't panic. Check the time of the month: the chances are that you will find you are starting your pre menstrual phase. Even if you put on weight, don't despair. Remember that this is only a temporary hiccup in your diet and it is not your fault. Your extra weight and size is water, not fat, and it will gradually melt away as your period starts. Accept a week of marking time, when you should be delighted if your weight stays the same and does not go up.

Eat sensibly even though you are on a diet. Don't be tempted to starve yourself or to miss out on vital foods. You need nourishment most at this time. But don't let that be the excuse to indulge with the thought, 'Oh well, I'm so fat today I might as well eat everything, tomorrow I'll starve!' That is the bad dieter's reasoning, because it provides the excuse for excessive eating today which you will only regret tomorrow.

Sometimes though it really is harder to stick to a diet during your pre menstrual days. You may find, for example, that you get food cravings when you are overwhelmed by desire for something sticky and sweet. The best way to deal with that is to **give in**, but in moderation. Go ahead and satisfy yourself with whatever it is you fancy – a couple of sweet biscuits, a glass of lemonade, a few squares of chocolate perhaps. But do not cheat and eat a whole packet of biscuits or two bars of chocolate. As we saw in Chapter One, one of the reasons for your craving may be a lowering of your blood sugar level. These sweet foods will have an immediate affect on that, but it will not last long. You need to eat more substantial foods, too, which are rich in nutrients and will nourish your body long-term. So, after you have nibbled your squares of chocolate, fill up with a slice of bread, a piece of cheese, a bowl of cereal or some raw carrots, or eat a good meal shortly afterwards.

If you are on a diet, and you feel horrified at the thought of eating bread, remember that it is a lot better for you, and much more likely to satisfy you, than a few squares of chocolate. And it is certainly a lot less fattening. Don't expect to stick rigidly to your diet all the time. None of us is perfect and when PMT strikes it can sap your will power. Indulge yourself sensibly as I have suggested and you should be able to mark time without bingeing. Then be glad that you have three good weeks coming up.

Exercise

Women have found some relief, particularly for their tension, by using relaxation and breathing exercises like those for expectant mothers.

One of the simplest is **3 stage breathing**, to help you breath calmly and easily when you feel tension mounting. Lie down flat on a bed, or better still on the floor, which is firmer, with a pillow under your head.

Stage One: breathe normally, breathing in through your nose and OUT through your mouth. Take your time. You should be taking about twelve breaths a minute.

Stage Two: breathe in and out through your mouth and nose together, and feel your ribcage move as you do so. Make the breath OUT stronger than the breath IN, so that you feel your lungs empty completely each time. You should be taking about twenty breaths a minute now.

Stage Three: breathe more quickly, less deeply now. Breathe IN naturally, say 'Ha' as you breathe OUT. You should be taking about forty breaths a minute now. Go through these stages gently and evenly, spending one minute on each level, or thirty seconds if you are feeling particularly tense, or if you have severe period pains. Follow the pattern of stage 1, 2, 3, 2, 1.

Another good exercise for relaxing the muscles of your womb and loosening tension in your shoulders or legs is **swimming**. If you cannot do the real thing, you can simulate it at home. Lie on a low table or stool, with a pillow under your stomach. Stretch your arms out in front of you and extend your legs. Now pretend that you are swimming breast stroke, and move your arms and legs slowly and firmly. Do this for two minutes, pause for a rest and then do it again. Three times in all once you have been exercising regularly.

Sometimes, specific exercises can help your aches and pains. A good **back exercise** is to lie flat on your back, feet together, arms by your sides and press the small of your back against the floor. Relax and then do this again, ten times. Tension often catches you in the neck and shoulder, so exercises like **neck swivels** may take away some of the stiffness. Starting with your head facing frontwards, shoulders down, arms relaxed by your sides, body upright,

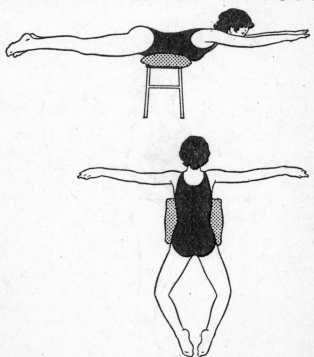

This swimming exercise may help to relieve your tension

rotate your head slowly from the front to the side to the back and to the side and back to the front again. Go round from right to left five times, then from left to right five times. Now tip your head backwards, straight, forwards, straight, sideways to the left, straight, sideways to the right, straight. Do this five times to each side. It is often helpful to do exercises like this to music, because it keeps you to a rhythm and makes them more fun.

For your **shoulders**, do simple arm swivels. Rotate your right arm ten times from front to back and then ten times

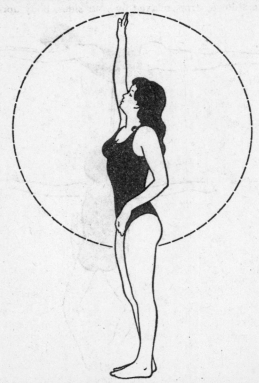

Arm swivels may help relieve tension in your neck and shoulders

from back to front. Do the same with your left arm. As with all exercises, you should start gradually. If you are too enthusiastic and overdo them at first, you will end up with more aches and pains, not less!

Some women have joined local yoga classes and found this a helpful way to relax. Some women swear by keep fit or dancing classes, because they feel that keeping their muscles in good shape seems to relieve some of their pain.

One trick to help you if you are feeling tense, is to lie down and concentrate on the part of you where the tension seems to have gathered – your neck, jaw, head, for instance. Think of it gradually relaxing. If it is your jaw that is tight, drop it open and then close it again without clenching your teeth. Move it from side to side. Loosen it. You may be surprised at how tightly clenched your teeth were, and how much better you feel now that you have noticed it and taken action.

If you get period pains, with cramps when your period starts (spasmodic dysmenorrhoea) then you may find that exercises bring you considerable relief. This is because, as we saw in Chapter Four, these pains are caused partly by the muscles of your womb contracting. Any exercises that use these muscles and relax them will help to relieve the pain. Two good books with ideas and exercises to help you are Hilary C. Maddux 'Menstruation' and Erna Wright 'Periods without Pain'.

Find your own favourite solution

We all have our own pet ways of coping with problems, and PMT should be no exception. Now that you know a bit more about PMT, pause to think of your own ways of making life easier during those days. To help you, here is an assorted selection of things that other women have found comforting and useful.

For the pain, whether aches and pains or period pains, the old-fashioned remedy of **heat** applied to the affected areas can be very soothing. There is a medical explanation for why this helps. Heat applied to muscles in spasm relaxes them and so eases the discomfort and accompanying pain. Try putting a hot water bottle where it hurts, or rub in a deep heating oil or cream. Some women take a hot bath and then lie down for a while. But be careful not to make the bath too hot as this could make you feel sick or faint.

Hot drinks, like tea, ordinary or herbal, or a nourishing soup, can warm and comfort you. But if you suffer from pre menstrual water retention, go easy on the quantity of liquid you drink.

Massage is another well known and much liked remedy, particularly for aching muscles, and tense neck and shoulders. Favourite, of course, is to get someone, preferably a professional, to do it for you. But failing that, give your neck and shoulders a going over yourself. Sit at a table, shoulders down, elbows resting lightly on the table. Put your hands round your neck and gently slide your fingers up and down your neck, pressing them into your skin as you go. First feel the bones in the centre of your neck. Then gradually move your hands apart and work up and down along the muscles in your neck.

Then, spread your fingers out and press them up under your hair, working your way from the bottom of your head right to the top and then across to your forehead and temples. Then put your right hand on your left shoulder and massage gently along the muscle, and do the same with your left hand on your right shoulder.

You could always combine this with some neck and arm swivels too. Your PMT won't suddenly evaporate, of course, but you might feel some relief.

Let off steam if you want to. It is no good bottling up your feelings. They will only come out in the end, probably more violently than you expected. If you feel tense and angry, retreat to your room and beat hell out of your pillow or buy or make a punch bag which you can pound. This may sound silly, but several women have told me that it works for them, and it is certainly better than kicking the cat, or taking it out on your family and friends.

Certain household tasks can be useful too. Sarah finds bread making a great relief: 'I slap and knead the dough so hard sometimes I don't think it can survive, but it certainly makes me feel better and seems to make better bread too!'

Susan washes clothes for the same reason: 'I think it is wringing them out that helps me most. It is a good way of relieving tension, and I can think of someone I don't like as I'm doing it!'

In the same way, if you feel like screaming, try to get away to somewhere where you can have a good scream. If you feel tearful, have a good cry. Some women have found that watching a sad film or reading a sad book provides the ideal excuse for a cry – and no one but you needs to know that you felt like crying anyway.

Reading, watching TV, or listening to music are all good ways of relaxing and taking your mind off your problems. Try to find an hour to sit down with a good book or watch a favourite programme. Many women find that an hour in bed reading or just listening to music before going to sleep, helps them get a good night's rest – and makes them feel stronger in the morning.

If you suffer from pre menstrual acne, or if your acne gets worse before your period, you could make a special effort to **avoid aggravating your spots.** Starting about 5 days before your PMT symptoms are due, wash your face carefully at least twice a day, using soap and water rather than a greasy make-up remover. Creams are the worst, but lotions also contain a fair amount of oil and grease and this is one of the main spot-causing culprits. Because of this, you should avoid grease wherever possible. Even if you usually use moisturiser, try leaving it off during this time. The same goes for foundation cream and powder. Try just using eye make-up or, if you must cover your face, try to find a water-based or grease-free make-up. As a last resort, a medicated cover stick may work, although the grease in it will probably outweigh the medication. Regular application of a good acne lotion is much more effective, and you should continue with it throughout the month, not just before your period, if your spots persist.

Painkilling drugs, like aspirin, may take the edge off your headache, though they are unlikely to banish it completely, and they sometimes help with aches and pains or menstrual cramps. There are also some drugs specially made to help with your period pains and also with PMT, which you can buy over the counter. It may be worth giving them a try to see if they bring you any relief.

To relieve tension, another possibility which is unusual but seems sometimes to be effective is sex. Masters and Johnson have shown that a woman's orgasm is a powerful means of relieving tension throughout the body at any time, and some women have found it particularly helpful when they are suffering from PMT. Even if, as we saw in Chapter Five, you find it hard to respond to your sexual partner at that time, or if he finds that you are not at your most appealing when irritable and depressed, it is worth talking it over with him. That way you can both try to see if you cannot be more loving at that time.

Being cuddled affectionately, or feeling the warmth of someone beside you, can be very comforting when you are feeling tense or miserable. And, if you reciprocate, it may convey better than words that, despite all appearances to the contrary during your pre menstrual days, you do still care for your partner.

Masturbation is another easy and good way to reach orgasm either alone or with a partner. Gradually, masturbation is being accepted as a normal part of our sexuality and some doctors, particularly those who specialise in sexual problems, recommend masturbation as a way of learning to reach orgasm so that it is easier to reach in intercourse. So don't be afraid of masturbation, the release of tension may actually help your PMT.

Some women have found that **acupuncture** has helped them. One London doctor found that some of her patients preferred acupuncture to more conventional forms of treatment for PMT. Of those who tried it, over three-quarters found acupuncture worked for them.

Another way to help your PMT is to **talk about it.** It is surprising how many women feel better once they know that they are not the only one who suffers, and discovering friends share your problems can make them easier to bear.

We made a television programme called 'Pull Yourself Together, Woman' some time ago, and received over 5000 letters, many of them from women who were simply delighted to find out that they were not alone.

'I thought, and so did my husband, that I was going mad. What a relief to know that I'm just like thousands of other women!'

Another wrote:

'I thought I had something terribly wrong with my breasts because they hurt so much sometimes. Then a friend mentioned that she had seen your programme and now she understood why her breasts swelled so much. We were both so relieved at the discovery that we stood giggling together like a couple of silly school children!'

Talking to other women and sharing ideas will probably give you other useful hints for how to cope. Talking to your husband, boyfriend, and children can make them understand you better and be more sympathetic. PMT is nothing to be ashamed of. The more it is discussed, the better it is understood. And that will help you – and every woman who suffers from PMT.

Look out for PMT in others

Once you have become aware of PMT in yourself, you will probably be able to see it more clearly in others. If you notice that friends of yours seem to get symptoms of PMT at about the same time each month, try gently bringing up the subject of PMT. They may not have heard of it, or have realised that it might be affecting them. Finding someone who shares their problems and can lend a sympathetic ear will be an enormous relief. And, of course, helping your friends to learn about treatment may banish their PMT for ever.

The same goes for your daughters. You may spot the beginnings of PMT long before they do, and helping them to come to terms with it and organise their lives to cope with it can be very useful. Sonia realised that her daughter Tessa played up at school and did not bother with her homework only at certain times each month. She noted the dates and found that there was a definite pattern connected with her daughter's periods. They talked it over and Tessa re-organised her homework as much as she could so that she never left herself extra work during that time and left as much as she could until she felt better. Sonia talked it over with Tessa's teachers, too, who were sympathetic and avoided confrontations with Tessa now they knew what was wrong. If your daughter's symptoms are severe, she may need treatment from the doctor. Spotting the signs early can save her – and you – a lot of misery later.

* * *

If you have tried the suggestions in this chapter and still feel you need more substantial treatment you should try to find an informed and sympathetic doctor who can help you. A doctor can guide you through treatment and check your progress, deciding with you which treatment is best for you and what dosage you need. The next chapter gives you details of the main treatments available and, as most of them are only obtainable on prescription, you will have to go to the doctor for them. The exception is Vitamin B6, which you can buy at most chemists. You will probably be better off having a doctor to help you with this treatment too but, if you really cannot find a doctor, you can find out in the next chapter how to use Vitamin B6 to treat yourself.

Help Yourself Reminder

PRIORITIES

1. Get organised for PMT.
2. Involve your family.
3. Eat sensibly.

THINGS TO TRY

1. Exercise
2. Heat treatment

3. Massage
4. Distractions
5. Sex
6. Acupuncture
7. Painkillers

Here are some books that you may find helpful:

DIET: WHAT TO EAT

Davis, Adele: **Let's Get Well**, Allen & Unwin, 1974
Yudkin, John: **This Nutrition Business**, Davis-Poynter, 1976

DIET: GENERAL

Edelstein, Barbara: **The Woman Doctor's Diet for Women,**
Prentice–Hall, 1977
Orbach, Susie: **Fat is a Feminist Issue,** Paddington Press,
1978

EXERCISE

Maddux, Hilary: **Menstruation**, Tobey Publishing Co., 1975
Noble, Elizabeth: **Essential Exercises for the childbearing
year**, John Murray Ltd., 1978
Wright, Erna: **Periods without Pain**, Tandem Books, 1975

Chapter Eleven

The Medical Solution

The good news is that even severe pre menstrual tension can be treated, and treated successfully. Now that doctors have worked out the physical reasons for PMT they can treat the root of the problem, instead of vainly trying to treat the symptoms. Proper treatment has dramatically relieved the discomforts of PMT, both physical and psychological, in well over three-quarters of women treated. That means that if you have PMT, the chances are very good indeed that you can be completely cured or helped so much that your symptoms are too mild to bother you any more.

The exact treatment you need depends on how severe your symptoms are. If you suffer only mildly you may be able to relieve many of your symptoms yourself (just follow the advice in Chapter Ten) or try Vitamin B6 (see page 130). On the other hand you may not want to take drugs, and are prepared to live with the discomforts of PMT, now you know why they occur. But if you suffer severely, then you probably need and want the doctor's help.

Family doctors know much more about PMT now than they did a few years ago, so your doctor should be sympathetic even if he is not sure what treatments are available. But there are some stick-in-the-mud doctors who refuse to believe in PMT and may try to fob you off with the wrong treatment or the wrong advice. Indeed, your doctor may have done this already, and you are reading this, desperately wondering what to do.

It might be a good idea to show your doctor this book. He can catch up on the facts, and he can follow up some of the medical references at the end of the book, and see the detailed medical research that has already been done. Some hospitals have now started PMT clinics in their Obstetrics and Gynaecology departments in order to study treatments further (see Appendix). Your doctor could find out if there is one in your area and refer you there for help.

If the worst comes to the worst, you could always change doctors. There are many who understand and sympathise with PMT sufferers and are only too willing to help. The treatments I mention are available almost worldwide, so with a few exceptions, you should be able to get whatever treatment you need. But in some countries the hormone therapy is used for treating other things, not PMT, so you will need to explain its use for your problem. Armed with this book, fight till you get the treatment you need!

*   *   *

One of the first things your doctor will ask you is what symptoms you have and when they occur. Look at the check-list of symptoms on Page 110 and mark the ones you suffer. Fill in the chart in Chapter Nine for two or three months and take it with you. If your symptoms are connected with your periods this will show up clearly on your chart.

The next step is diagnosis. As we said in Chapter Three the cause of PMT can be either a hormone imbalance, with a deficiency of progesterone, or a deficiency of pyridoxine, (vitamin B6). Your symptoms may be a guide to which particular deficiency is your problem but, without sophisticated radioimmunoassay techniques, it is sometimes very hard to tell. Some doctors, therefore, prefer to try the mildest treatment, vitamin B6, first and only progress to hormone treatment if that does not work.

If you suffer from symptoms like migraine, asthma or epilepsy, which you do get anyway, but which get worse pre menstrually, one bonus of treating your PMT will be that, under medical supervision, you can reduce the medicine you take for these symptoms during the rest of the month.

The reason for this is that your treatment is based on your worst attacks, which occur before your period. Once these have been lightened, you can go on to less powerful drugs, or a smaller dosage, to control your less serious attacks at other times of the month. Doctors at St Thomas's Hospital found that, for women with epilepsy, for example, they could reduce their anticonvulsant drugs by one third after treating the women for PMT.

Vitamin B6

Pyridoxine, also known as Vitamin B6, is the mildest and simplest of treatments. It is available without prescription from most chemists because it is not a drug, but a vitamin. It is already present to some extent naturally in your body, and is a water-soluble vitamin, like Vitamin C, so that taking extra will not do you any harm because any excess will be excreted with your urine. (Incidentally, this is not true of other vitamins, which can be stored in the body and so should not be taken in large amounts.) If your doctor is really unsympathetic you could try this treatment for yourself.

You should start taking Vitamin B6 three days before your symptoms are due to start, which will probably be about ten days before your period, and continue taking it until three days after your period has started, roughly thirteen or fourteen days each month. Most women start with a dosage of 20 milligrams twice a day, morning and evening, making a total of 40 milligrams each day, but if you find that that does not seem to have much effect, you should try a slightly higher dose next time, say 40 milligrams twice a day, or a total of 80 milligrams a day.

Do not be discouraged if there does not seem to be any improvement right away. Vitamin B6 deficiency is strange in that there is not necessarily a gradual improvement as you top up your vitamin level: you will probably only see and feel an improvement when you reach the right dosage. That is where a skilful doctor could help by gauging more accurately what amount of Vitamin B6 you need. It is definitely worth persevering with gradually higher doses if you do not succeed at first, because you may suddenly hit on the right amount and be wonderfully relieved of most or all of your symptoms. However, you should never take more than 200 milligrams of Vitamin B6 a day, because more than that can cause unpleasant gastric acidity. If such a high dose does not work for you, you obviously need a different treatment.

Generally you should continue treatment for about nine months and many women find their symptoms never recur. But, if you do start suffering again, you can safely restart treatment and continue taking Vitamin B6 each month at the crucial time.

Sometimes doctors have had remarkable success with Vitamin B6. Professor P. H. F. Giles of Perth in Australia was one of the first to use pyridoxine for PMT and he has had very good results with it. At St Thomas's Hospital in London, over 80% of women with pre menstrual headaches were completely cured, and nearly two thirds (65%) of the women suffering from PMT generally were either completely cured or very much improved.

'Since I started taking Vitamin B6 I'm like a different person. No more headaches, no more aggression. Just *me* all the time, which is a wonderful experience.'

'It is absolutely marvellous to have no depression. I can hardly believe each month comes and goes without any ups and downs. It seems impossible now that I ever felt as unbalanced as I used to.'

Recent research indicates that Vitamin B6 may also be able to help you with **menopause.** (Menopause is a large subject on its own, and is outside the scope of this book.) If you are approaching the menopause, and are starting to find that your periods are becoming increasingly scanty and irregular, you may have started to suffer some of the symptoms of the menopause.

St Thomas's Hospital have found that a dose of 10 or 20 milligrams of Vitamin B6 taken every day can help relieve some of the early symptoms of the menopause and make the transition period less distressing. Very little research has been done on this yet, but as the vitamin cannot do you any harm, and it might do you a considerable amount of good, it certainly seems worth a try.

Dydrogesterone

Dydrogesterone is a progestogen, the name given to a synthetic version of the hormone progesterone. You will remember from Chapter Three, that PMT often appears to be caused by a deficiency in the level of progesterone in your blood at a crucial time in your menstrual cycle, or by imbalance between your oestrogen and progesterone levels. If this is your problem, the level of progesterone in your blood needs to be topped up: this is where dydrogesterone comes in.

There are various different progestogens, but dydrogesterone is the one that most closely resembles natural progesterone, and has been found to be most successful when used to treat PMT. St Thomas's Hospital in London, for instance, found that nearly three-quarters of all the women they treated with dydrogesterone were completely cured or were so much better that they were easily able to cope with any symptoms that remained. In particular, most women found that their psychological symptoms were greatly relieved, and almost all were cured of their water retention.

One extreme example of this was a woman who suffered so badly from water retention that her ankles and legs used to swell enormously and she put on at least 14lbs regularly in the week before her period. After treatment with dydrogesterone, her swelling and extra weight disappeared completely. And in France, Mauvais-Jarvis and J. P. Bercovici, who have been using dydrogesterone for over six years, found a spectacular improvement in 80% of the women they treated for PMT.

Dydrogesterone is marketed under the name Duphaston,

and comes in the form of tablets to be swallowed. It is only available on prescription so you have to go to a doctor for this treatment. The usual dose you start with is 10 milligrams twice a day; making 20 milligrams a day in all, from Days 12 to 26 of your cycle (Day 1 being the first day of your period). If this dose does not work, the doctor might increase it to 40 milligrams a day, or very occasionally even more, and then gradually reduce the amount you take as your symptoms improve.

As with pyridoxine, treatment usually lasts from six to nine months but if your symptoms come back when you've stopped taking the tablets you can continue with the treatment for longer.

So far, dydrogesterone has very few side effects. About 5% of women taking it under supervision at St Thomas's Hospital suffered minor effects like mild nausea, increased breast tenderness, or new breast tenderness which they had not had before. Occasionally, some women have found that they get slight changes in their menstrual cycle. But apart from these, no other side effects have been found.

With any hormone tablet, there is often a worry about whether or not it can cause cancer. In all the tests that have been done with dydrogesterone there has been absolutely no evidence uncovered that suggests it has any cancer causing effect. In fact, dydrogesterone is actually used in the treatment of certain forms of cancer.

'Since taking the hormone tablets the change is quite amazing. I no longer feel depressed or aggressive nor do my fingers or breasts feel uncomfortably swollen. In fact, there is now no difference in the way I feel before a period to the rest of the month. I am astonished that something which has been going on so long can vanish completely and so quickly.'

'I am now able to report after two cycles of dydrogesterone, there is a marked improvement. I experienced no feelings of lethargy and was particularly pleased to find that I did not feel weepy or irritable – my improved temper was noticed by my husband. During my last cycle, I was under some pressure at work and at home and coped with this quite adequately, which would not have been the case before this treatment. I can sum up by saying that during the second half of my cycle I felt as I normally do during the first half.'

Natural Progesterone

The natural hormone, progesterone, was first extracted from the ovaries of certain animals, but this was a difficult process and supplies were limited. In 1943, it was found that it could be manufactured from the roots of yams, and was used a great deal as the basis for the manufacture of other hormones, like cortisone and some synthetic progesterones such as those used in the contraceptive pill. For some years this has been its main use but, because it is identical with the progesterone that occurs naturally in women, it is also used in the treatment of PMT.

You may be wondering why, if it is the same as natural progesterone, it is not the favourite treatment for PMT. The problem with it is that it cannot be taken by mouth because it is broken down too quickly in the gut and by the liver on the way to general circulation round the body. This means that you have to take it either as an injection or as suppositories or pessaries, which are inserted in the vagina or rectum. These are not particularly attractive methods of treatment compared with a simple pill, and from a practical point of view, treatment with natural progesterone is much more expensive than either dydrogesterone or Vitamin B6. For all these reasons, doctors have been reluctant to prescribe natural progesterone, and the comparatively recent discovery of dydrogesterone has been a breakthrough for the treatment of PMT.

But if neither Vitamin B6 nor dydrogesterone work for you, maybe natural progesterone will. Many women have found it very successful and feel that it is worth the effort of an injection or suppositories to be free of their symptoms.

Again, progesterone is only available on prescription, and it is really up to you and your doctor to decide how much you need. An average dose is 400 milligrams a day but some women find they need as much as four times that amount a day at their worst. Usually you start taking progesterone four or five days before your symptoms are due to start and continue until your period begins, or until your symptoms would normally disappear anyway. Some doctors allow their patients a certain flexibility, so that you can take an extra suppository if your symptoms are particularly severe and you are not getting sufficient relief from your normal dose.

If you have already had a child you can probably tolerate very high levels of progesterone because, during pregnancy, you will already have experienced very high progesterone levels manufactured by the placenta to nourish your growing baby. But if you have not had children, you may find that if you take too much progesterone, you become euphoric, with excessive restless energy so that you cannot sleep, or you may get cramps rather like spasmodic dysmenorrhoea during your periods. If you do experience any of these symptoms, you should reduce the amount of progesterone you take.

In 30 years, no serious side effects have been found. There may be small changes in your menstrual cycle and if you take large doses you may find that your periods stop altogether until you stop treatment or reduce your dosage. As with dydrogesterone, there is no indication at all that progesterone can cause cancer and it, too, is used in the treatment of certain forms of cancer.

'Since taking progesterone I feel that I am in control of myself for the first time in fourteen years. No more tempers, no more crying fits for no reason, no more awful depressions. My husband cannot believe the change – he keeps saying, "Now I've got back the woman I married!"'

'I think my marriage was saved by receiving progesterone treatment, and I am certain that my children are much calmer and happier than they used to be. Well, it is hardly surprising really. I used to be a terrible wife and mother for two weeks out of four, but now I find I can cope even under pressure. I have gone back to work too, something I never dared contemplate before.'

Bromocryptine

Bromocryptine is a fairly new drug available only on prescription, which has the effect of lowering an excessively high level of prolactin in the blood. In Holland doctors have had some success in treating PMT with bromocryptine but trials in Britain have so far proved less promising. St Thomas's Hospital, for instance, found that it is useful for women who suffer from very painful breasts and that it can, occasionally, help with other symptoms. But they only use it as a last resort because the success rate with it has not been very high, it is a very powerful drug and some women get unpleasant side effects like nausea, or lowered blood pressure or minor visual symptoms. It is possible, though, that as more is found out about the effects of a raised prolactin level, bromocryptine may be more effectively used.

* * *

Over 80% of women who suffer PMT severely have found enormous relief with the treatments I have outlined. For some, they have only succeeded in giving partial relief. Occasionally specialist PMT clinics may use other unusual and sometimes very powerful drugs to deal with one or more very stubborn problems. Research continues, and as more is understood about the causes of PMT, new treatments will be found.

* * *

The treatments that we have mentioned are the newest and most effective for PMT. Others have been tried with less success. In particular, the following may have been suggested to you.

Diuretics

Diuretics are tablets that help to speed up water loss from your tissues. If you have very mild PMT, where bloating is your biggest problem, they may be helpful. But if your PMT is more serious, they will not be very effective because the problem is more fundamental – most of your symptoms are caused by hormone imbalance or a need for Vitamin B6, and not by excessive water retention.

It is rather like trying to dry out dampness in your walls with an electric fire instead of a damp proof course. The damp will keep coming back, because you are not touching the cause of the problem. In the same way, water will continue to build up in your cells, and you will keep on having to take diuretics to get rid of it. If you use diuretics too much, they can upset your potassium and sodium levels, which can make your PMT worse. Diuretics are available on prescription only, so in any case you will require a doctor's approval. Be sure that you tell your doctor you think that your bloatedness is related to PMT.

Tranquillisers

Many women are given tranquillisers when they go to their doctor with the symptoms of PMT. Usually this is because the doctor does not realise that the symptoms are connected with PMT, or because he simply does not know what other treatments are available.

Tranquillisers are **not** a treatment for PMT. If you are very anxious and tense they may reduce these feelings but, because they are cerebral depressants, they may make you feel dopey, lethargic and depressed too. If these are already symptoms you are suffering because of PMT, you will simply feel worse. Many women have found this out the hard way but carry on taking tranquillisers because they do not know what else to do.

If your doctor has prescribed tranquillisers for you, but your menstrual chart shows a clear connection between your

137

symptoms and your periods, you should talk to him about switching to one of the treatments in this book.

The contraceptive pill

There is often confusion about the role of the contraceptive pill: does it or does it not help with PMT?

The contraceptive pill is composed of synthetic hormones, usually a combination of oestrogens and progestogens. As we saw, progestogen is the name given to synthetic progesterone-like substances and the two types should not be confused, though unfortunately even some doctors do muddle the two. There are many different progestogens, some of which resemble natural progesterone more than others. Dydrogesterone is so similar to natural progesterone that it is one of the best, and most successful forms of treatment for PMT. (And, incidentally, it does **not** have a contraceptive effect, so that you can still get pregnant while taking it.) Other progestogens, however, which are used in different contraceptive pills, depending on the brand, may have some of the beneficial effects of progesterone. But they may also have unpleasant side effects that progesterone does not have.

You may find that, once you have found a pill that suits you, it does help relieve your PMT. This may be, in part, because the contraceptive pill stops ovulation, and women who do not ovulate rarely if ever suffer from PMT. Or it may be because the Pill suppresses your normal hormonal ups and downs and replaces them with a constant level of oestrogen and progesterone.

But there are some women who get many of the symptoms of PMT while on the Pill, especially depression. And, of course, there are a variety of side effects with the Pill which many women do not want to risk.

So the contraceptive pill is not necessarily a satisfactory treatment for PMT. If you want to use the Pill as a contraceptive anyway you may be able to find one that helps you. But otherwise you would be much better off trying one of the other treatments.

Conclusion

Looking Forward

This book has brought you up-to-date with the latest research on the causes of PMT, and outlined the treatments available. I hope that we have stripped PMT of its mystery – and brought it out in the open so that you can talk about it freely, without fear of ridicule.

The future looks bright. Things should get better and better for PMT sufferers. Now that PMT is firmly established as a real physical problem, more research is being done into its causes. New discoveries are being made all the time. As a result, new treatments are sure to be found.

Most important of all, attitudes to PMT are changing. People in general are much more sympathetic and understanding towards women who suffer, and you are unlikely to be doped with tranquillisers and sent away as 'neurotic' when you go to your doctor for help.

Indeed, you can help people to understand PMT as well. If we talk about it openly, sympathise and help others, and help ourselves, then we can make sure that the problem of PMT is treated with the respect it deserves.

You can help us too. We will be updating this book as soon as we hear of new research or developments in the treatment of PMT. If you have any ideas that you would like to share with other women – suggestions, tips, advice, things to do or not to do for coping with PMT – please let us know. We will be delighted to include your ideas in the next edition of this book.

The address to write to is:

PMT
c/o Melbourne House Publishers
24 Red Lion Street
London WC1
England

References

Chapter One

P 20f *Premenstrual Tension*, Dr E. Trimmer, B.J.S.M., April 1979.

P 20 Diamond, S. *et al:* Menstrual Problems in Women with Primary Affective Illness, *Comprehensive Psych*, 17 541–48 1976.
Dr Clare's research is reported in *Current Medical Research and Opinion*, Vol. 4. Suppl. 4, 1977 and in *Current Medical Research and Opinion* Vol. 6, Suppl. 5, 1979.

P 24 Low blood sugar see Billig, H. E. & Spaulding, C. A.: *Ind. Medicine* 16, 336, 1947. Dalton, K.: *The Premenstrual Syndrome and Progesterone Therapy*, Heinemann Medical Books, 1977.

P 29 For studies mentioned, see references for Chapter Seven.

P 30 Dalton, K.: 'Influence of Menstruation on Glaucoma', *British Journal of Ophthalmology*, 1967, 51, 10, 692–95.

Chapter Three

P 42f Many books discuss the basic mechanisms of the menstrual cycle. One example is, Taylor & Brush, *Concise Medical Text of Obstetrics and Gynaecology*, Bailliere, 1978.

Calt, K. J.: *ABC of Endocrinology*, published by Lancet, 1971.

P 47   Frank, R. T.: *Arch. Neurol. Psych.*, 26, 1053 1931. Israel: *J.A.M.A.*, 110, 1721, 1938.

P 48   Studies on hormonal imbalance conducted at St Thomas's Hospital, London are reported in *Current Medical Research and Opinion*, Vol. 4, Suppl. 4, 1977 and Vol. 6, Suppl. 5, 1979.
Munday, M. R. *et al: Journal Endocrinology*, 73, 21, 1977.
Backstrom, T. & Carstensen, H.: *Journ. Steroid Biochemistry*, 5, 257, 1974.

P 55f   Dysmenorrhoea, see Taylor & Brush, *Concise Medical Text of Obstetrics and Gynaecology*, Bailliere, 1978.

Chapter Four

P 57f   Moos, R. H.: *Menstrual Distress Questionnaire Manual*, Stanford University, California, 1977.

P 58f   Not enough research has been done in this area and, to be fair, some studies take a view opposed to mine. Studies dealing with the topic include: Shainess, N.: A re-evaluation of some aspects of femininity through a study of menstruation: a preliminary report, *Comprehensive Psychiatry* 2: 20–26, 1961; Behrman, S. J. & Gosling, J. R.: *Fundamentals of Gynaecology*, Second Edition. Oxford University Press, New York, 1966; Rubele, D. *et al:* research on menstrual related psychological changes. Alternative perspectives. *Paper published at the conference on bio-psychological factors influencing sex-role related behaviours, Smith College, Northampton, Mass., October 1976.* Paige, K.: Women learn to sing the menstrual blues, *Psychology Today* (USA), 4: 41–46, 1973.

P 58f   Nicholson, J.: *A Question of Sex*, Fontana, 1979.

P 59   Quotation from the television programme, 'All in the Family', written by Michael Ross and Bernie West, copyright 1973, Tandem Productions Inc.

P 63   Paige, K.: Effects of oral contraceptives on affective fluctuations associated with the menstrual cycle: *Psychosomatic Medicine*, 33 (6), 515–537, 1971.

Chapter Five

P 68   Research by Roger Langley and Richard Levy is quoted in *Once A Month* by K. Dalton, Fontana, 1978.

Chapter Six

P 76   Surgery attendance of mothers with sick children: *The Menstrual Cycle*, Dalton, K., Penguin Books.
Children's hospital admissions related to mothers' menstrual cycle, Dalton, K.: *Lancet* 11, 1386, 1968.

P 94   Story of Susan taken from Dalton, K., *Once A Month*, Fontana, 1978.

Chapter Seven

P 84f   A good overview of research on reflexes, concentration, etc., is Summer, B.: The effect of menstruation on Cognitive and Perceptual-Motor Behaviour: A Review, *Psychosomatic Medicine*, 35 (6), 1973.
Baisdon, A. and Gibson, R.: Effects of the Menstrual Cycle on Performance of Complex Perceptual-Psychomotor Tasks. *Paper to Human Factors Society*, Dallas, Texas, 1975.

P 87   I mention *Menstruation and Menopause* by Paula Weideger, published by Knopf, N.Y., 1975.

P 88   Research on schoolgirls' examinations is from Dalton, K.: 'O' level failures in relation to girls' menstrual cycle: *Lancet*, 11, 1386, 1968.

P 90   Accident statistics from engineering factories, hospitals and doctors' surgeries admissions are from an unpublished report to the *Medical Commission on Accident Prevention*, by Dr Patricia Lees: The Vulnerability to Trauma of Women in relation to Periodic Stress.
Survey of accident admissions to hospitals is by Dalton, K.: *British Medical Journal*, 2, 1425, 1960.

P 92   Research on women and crime includes: Dalton, K., Timing of women's offences during the menstrual cycle: *British Medical Journal*, 2, 1752, 1961; Morton *et al*, A clinical study of Pre Menstrual Tension: *American Journal of Obstetrics and Gynaecology*, 65, 1182–1191, 1953.

P 93f   The studies from which my information is taken are:
         Zaharieva, E. J., Survey of sportswomen at the Tokyo
         Olympics, *Journal Sports Med. Phys. Fitness*, 5, 215,
         1965; Wearing, M. P. *et al*, The effects of the men-
         strual cycle on tests of physical fitness, *Journ. Sports
         Med. Phys. Fitness*, 12, 38, 1972; Zimmerman, E.
         and Parlee, M. B.: Behavioural changes associated
         with the menstrual cycle, *Journ. Appl. Soc. Psychol.*,
         3, 4335, 1972; Loucks, J. and Thompson H.: Effects
         of menstruation on reaction time: *Res. Q. Am. Ass.
         Hlth. Phys. Fitness*, 39, 2, 407, 1968.

Chapter Eight

P 97f   Brown, G. W. and Harris, T.: *Social Origins of De-
         pression*, Tavistock, 1968.
P 100   Survey on alcoholism in U.S.A., Belfen, M. L. and
         Carroll, M.: *Arch. Gen. Psychiat.*, 25, 240, 1971.
P 101f   There have been several surveys on suicide and
         suicide attempts in relation to PMT. Some of them
         are: Tonks, C. M. *et al*, Attempted suicide and the
         menstrual cycle: *Journal Psychosomatic Research*, 2,
         319, 1968: Glass *et al*, Psychiatric emergency related
         to the menstrual cycle, *American Jour. Psychiatry*,
         128, 705–711, 1971; Mandell and Mandell, Suicide and
         the menstrual cycle, *Journ. American Medical Assoc.*,
         200, 792–3, 1967; Lees, Dr P.: The vulnerability to
         trauma of women in relation to periodic stress. Un-
         published report to the *Medical Commission on Acci-
         dent Prevention*; MacKinnon and MacKinnon, Lethal
         hazards of the luteal phase of the menstrual cycle;
         British Medical Journal, 1, 1015–1017, 1959.

Chapter Nine

P 110   Our symptoms checklist is based on, Moos, R. H.:
         Menstrual Distress Questionnaire, Stanford Univer-
         sity, California, 1977.

Chapter Ten

P 118f   Adapted from Wright, E.: *Periods Without Pain*, Tan-
         dem Books, 1975.

P 124   Masters, W. H. and Johnson, V. E.: *Human Sexual Response*, Little Brown, 1966.

Chapter Eleven

P 130f   Kerr, G. D.: *Current Medical Opinion and Research*, Suppl. 4, 29, 1977. A placebo controlled trial of pyridoxine in PMT carried out at St Thomas's Hospital has been completed and will be published by Day, *et al.*

P 131   Reitz, R.: *Menopause, A Positive Approach*, Harvester, 1979.

P 132f   Various studies have examined the safety of dydrogesterone. The main ones are: Villedieu, P. and Mousselon, J.: *Presse Med*, 71, 337, 1963; Barnard, I.: *Gynae. Pract. XIII*, 477–496, 1962; Boris, A., *et al: Steroids*, 7, 1–10, 1966; Greenblatt, R. B.: *Third World Congress of Gynae and Obstet.*, Vienna, Austria, 1961; Vermylen, J., *et al: Journ. Obstet. Gynaec. Brit. Commonwealth*, 80, 75–81, 1973; Aydar, C. K. and Greenblatt, R. B.: *Int. Journ. Fertility IX*, 585–595, 1964; Becker, M. H.: *Obstet. and Gynaec.*, 19, 724–729, 1962; Marois, M.: *Bull. Acad. Nat. Med.*, 146, 324–334, 349–364, 1962; Scholer, H. F. L.: Lecture to Royal Society Med. on Actions and uses of Orally Active Progestational Steroids, 1962.
There is a large amount of literature on the use of progestogens in the treatment of endometrial cancer. The following give a number of papers and reviews on the subject. Brush, M. G., Taylor R. W. & Williams, D. C.: *Symposium on Endometrial Caneer*, Heinnemann, 1973; Brush, M. G. & Taylor, R. W. (Eds.): *Gynaecological Malignancy, Clinical and Experimental Studies*, Bailliere, 1975; Brush, M. G., King, R. J. B. & Taylor, R. W. (Eds.): *Endometrial Cancer*, Bailliere, 1978.

P 132   Taylor, R. W.: *Current Medical Opinion and Research* 4, Suppl. 4, 35, 1977. A placebo controlled trial of Dydrogesterone in PMT carried out at St Thomas's Hospital will shortly be published by Kerr, *et al.*

P 132   Mauvais-Jarvis, P. and Bercovici, J. P.: The place of 6-Dehydro-retroprogesterone in Endocrine Gynaecology, *Gaz. Med. Fr.*, 76, 2551–2555, 1969.

P 134f   Dalton, K.: *The Premenstrual Syndrome and Proges-terone Therapy*, Heinemann Medical Books, 1977.

P 138   Gunn, A. D. G.: *British Journal of Sexual Medicine*, 3, 4, 14, 1976.

Bromocryptine:

P 136   Benedeh-Jaszmann & Hearn-Startevant, *Lancet* **i**, 1095, 1976.
            Anderson, *et al: Brit. Journ. Obstet. Gynaec.*, 84, 370, 1977.
            Andersch, *et al: Acta Endocrin.*, 88, Suppl. 1, 165, 1978.

Illustration References

Chapter One

Time of physical symptoms in survey of 500 women: Kessel, N. & Coppen, A., *Lancet*, 2, 61, 1963.

Chapter Two

Time of psychological symptoms in survey of 500 women: *op cit.*

Chapter Three

Comparison between the level of progesterone in a normal woman and one suffering from pre menstrual tension: Figure 1. Munday, M. R.: *Current Medical Research and Opinion*, Vol. 4, Suppl. 4, 1977.

Chapter Six

Surgery attendance of mothers with sick children: *The Menstrual Cycle*, Dalton, K., Penguin Books.
Children's hospital admissions related to mothers' menstrual cycle, Dalton, K., *Lancet*, 11, 1386, 1968.

Chapter Seven

Comparative statistics for attendances at doctors' surgeries, hospital admissions, accidents in general and car accidents are taken from an unpublished report by the Medical Committee on Accident Prevention.

Timing of women's offences during menstrual cycle: Dalton, K., *BMJ*, 2, 1752, 1961.

Chapter Eight

Taken from Dalton, K., *The Premenstrual Syndrome and Progesterone Therapy*, Heinemann Medical Books, 1977.

Bibliography

Brush, M. G.: *Pre Menstrual Tension and Period Pains*, Women's Health Concern, 1979.

Dalton, K.: *The Premenstrual Syndrome and Progesterone Therapy*, Heinemann Medical Books, 1977.

Dalton, K.: *Once A Month*, Fontana Paperbacks, 1978.

Delaney, *et al*: *The Curse*, Mentor Books, 1977.

Shuttle, P. & Redgrove, P.: *The Wise Wound*, Richard Marek Publishers, 1978.

Weideger, Paula: *Menstruation and Menopause*, Delta Books, Dell Publishing Co. Inc., 1977.

Migraine

Sacks, O.: *Migraine, Evolution of a Common Disorder*, Faber & Faber, 1973.

Diet

Davis, Adele: *Let's Get Well*, Unwin Paperbacks, 1966.

Edelstein, Barbara: *The Woman Doctor's Diet*, Prentice-Hall Inc., 1977.

Orbach, Susie: *Fat is a Feminist Issue*, Paddington Press, 1978.

Yudkin, John: *This Nutrition Business*, Davis Poynter, 1976.

Exercise

Maddux, Hilary: *Menstruation*, Tobey Publishing Co., 1975.
Wright, Erna: *Periods Without Pain*, Tandem, 1966.

Index

152

153

Appendix

Where to get help

Obviously one of the first people to go to for help is your local GP. But if he is unable or unwilling to treat you there are several other places to try.

There are four hospitals in Britain which run special PMT clinics. These are:

Chelsea Hospital for Women
Dovehouse Street
London SW3

Hallamshire Hospital
Sheffield

St Thomas's Hospital
Lambeth Palace Road
London SE1

A leaflet on Vitamin B6 treatment can be obtained by sending an s.a.e. to PMT Clinic, Gynaecology Dept., St Thomas's Hospital, London SE1.

University College Hospital
Gower Street
London WC1

There is also one small private clinic in London:

Marie Stopes Clinic
The Wellwoman Centre
108 Whitfield Street
London W1

Apart from these specialist clinics, there are a number of organisations which may be able to help you.

The Women's Health Concern
16 Seymour Street
London W1

Family Planning Clinics – these are run by the NHS and can be found in most towns throughout Britain (look in your local telephone directory for the address and telephone number of the one nearest you). They may be able to tell you the nearest clinic or hospital which treats PMT.

The Family Planning Information Service
27 Mortimer Street
London NW1
Tel: 01–636 7866

You can ring or write to them for information on a PMT treatment centre in your area.

The Citizens' Advice Bureau – there are Citizens' Advice Bureaus in most towns throughout Britain (see your local telephone directory). They can put you in touch with the nearest clinic or hospital which treats PMT.

The Marriage Guidance Council – there are Marriage Guidance Council branches in most towns throughout Britain (see your local telephone directory). They are skilled at dealing with all sorts of marital problems, including those caused by PMT, and should be able to give you advice and help. If you have difficulty finding a local branch you can write or ring:

The London Marriage Guidance Council
76a New Cavendish Street
London W1
Tel: 01–580 1087

Migraine Trust
45 Great Ormond Street
London W1

If you suffer from migraine you can contact the Trust for advice and information.

Alcoholics Anonymous – there are branches of Alcoholics Anonymous in most towns (see your local telephone directory). If you have a drinking problem and want help you could join one of their groups. If you have difficulty finding a local branch you can write for information to:

Alcoholics Anonymous
PO Box 514
11 Redcliffe Gardens
London SW10 9BG

Accept
Western Hospital
Seagrave Road
London SW6
Tel: 01–381 3155

ACCEPT is a treatment centre for people with drinking problems. They hold regular group sessions to make women more aware of the pressures of PMT and its relationship to excessive drinking.

The Women's Therapy Centre
6 Manor Gardens
London N7 6LA

The Women's Therapy Centre holds regular therapy sessions for women with psychological problems. If you feel that the treatments we suggest are not sufficient on their own, you may find help and advice at the Women's Therapy Centre.

The Samaritans – The Samaritans have branches and a night and day telephone service in most towns in Britain (see your local telephone directory) to help people who are feeling desperate, depressed or suicidal. If you cannot find a branch in your area you can write for help to:

The Samaritans
39 Walbrook
London EC4

About the Authors

JUDY LEVER is a journalist who worked for IPC magazines and is currently a Producer/Director with Thames Television. In this capacity, she was the producer of the Thames Television programme on Pre Menstrual Tension entitled 'Pull Yourself Together, Woman'. She is currently working on another book.

DR MICHAEL G. BRUSH has specialised in medical endocrinology since 1968 in the post of Senior Lecturer for Biochemistry in the Dept. of Gynaecology at St Thomas's Hospital Medical School, London.

His research in Pre Menstrual Tension has led him to discover progesterone deficiencies and vitamin losses in women who suffer PMT. This research resulted in the formation of the first clinic for hormone testing for Pre Menstrual sufferers.

Dr Brush has published over 50 research papers and in 1977 he contributed a paper on the mechanisms causing PMT in 'Current Medical Research and Opinion'.

His previous books have included 'The Concise Medical Text – Obstetrics and Gynaecology' (Co-author Prof. R. W. Taylor) and three volumes on Gynaecological Cancer. (Co-editor).

BRIAN HAYNES is a former *Sunday Times* journalist who now works in the Current Affairs department of Thames Television. He has co-authored a thriller called 'Spyship'. (Allen Lane).